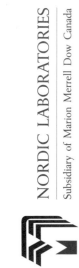

NORDIC LABORATORIES

Subsidiary of Marion Merrell Dow Canada

2150 St. Elzear Blvd. W.
Laval, Quebec H7L 4A8
Telephone: (514) 331-9220
Fax: (514) 334-8016

May 1994

Dear Doctor,

Nordic Laboratories Inc., a subsidiary of Marion Merrell Dow (Canada) Inc., is pleased to announce it is launching a new program designed especially for physicians across Canada. *Heartmates®, A Survival Guide for the Cardiac Spouse*, an acclaimed book for cardiac families, is now available to you for your patients. Enclosed is a complimentary copy of this informative book for your perusal.

This patient education resource is part of *Heartmates®*, the first hospital-affiliated program designed to meet the psycho-social needs of spouses and patients with heart disease. These resources have been reviewed by the Canadian Cardiovascular Society and the Canadian Association of Cardiac Rehabilitation, and have received their endorsement as a useful adjunct in the management of heart disease.

Heartmates®, A Survival Guide for the Cardiac Spouse, was designed to complement the professional counsel you offer your patients. Authored by Rhoda Levin, a clinical social worker by profession, the book was inspired by her personal experience with this devastating disease, as her husband survived two heart attacks and bypass surgery. The book examines and explains in lay language the psychological implications (anxiety, grief, loss of old lifestyle) of heart disease for patients as well as family members. It also addresses issues most frequently encountered in the office-based practice relating to lifestyle changes, overprotective behaviour, fears concerning sexual activity and the recovery process.

If you are interested in receiving this program, you will be sent eight complimentary copies of *Heartmates*® to give to your patients. A re-order form will be included if you wish to obtain additional copies of the book. The books are packaged in a practical bookholder for easy access, along with a directory of all hospitals and institutions across Canada that utilize other *Heartmates*® resources, such as the five video programs for patients and their families. This listing will assist you in patient referrals.

We hope the books will be a useful adjunct in addressing the needs of your patients and their families. We look forward to continuing to work with you to provide these resources to those who need them.

Simply fill out the enclosed Business Reply Card to receive your complimentary copies of *Heartmates*®, while supplies last. Nordic Laboratories is proud to present this program to physicians, as part of our continuing education service.

Sincerely,

Melanie Anonychuk
Product Manager, Cardizem
Nordic Laboratories Inc.

®Heartmates is a registered trademark of Heartmates Inc., Minneapolis, Minnesota U.S.A.

Heartmates®

A Survival Guide
for the
Cardiac Spouse

Rhoda F. Levin

FOREWORD BY

David V. Keith, M.D.
Director of Family Therapy
State University of New York, Syracuse

MinervaPress
A Division of the J.D. Scram Company
Minneapolis, Minnesota, U.S.A.

Heartmates® A Survival Guide For The Cardiac Spouse
Copyright © 1987 by Rhoda F. Levin

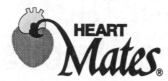

Heartmates® is a registered trademark of Heartmates, Inc.

All rights reserved. Inquiries about the use of the material in this book
should be addressed to: Permissions, MinervaPress, a division of the
J.D. Scram Company, P.O. Box 16202, Minneapolis, MN 55416.

Library of Congress Cataloging-in-Publication Data

Levin, Rhoda F.
    Heartmates® A Survival Guide For The Cardiac Spouse

    Bibliography: p.
    Includes index.
    1. Heart — Infarction — Patients — Family relationships.
    2. Wives   I. Title
    RC685.I6L43   362.1'961237   87-11392
ISBN 0-9637795-0-8
(previously published by Prentice Hall Press, ISBN 0-13-385162-1)

Cover and interior design: Cottage Communications
Cover art: "Fields of Choice" © 1994 by Bonnie S. Barland
Author's photograph © 1992 by Larry Marcus

This edition is printed on an acid-free paper that meets the American
National Standards Institute Z39.48 Standard.

Manufactured in the U.S.A.

10 9 8 7 6 5 4 3 2 1

I dedicate this book to my husband, Marsh,
who is my heartmate;
and to our children, Sidney and Deborah,
and to their children's children.

ACKNOWLEDGMENTS

There are many people, here unnamed, who have contributed to my growth and in some way have made this book possible. I am grateful to all of them: those I have worked with as colleagues and clients, those I have known personally, and those who have taught me through their writing. I thank each and all of them. I am especially grateful to:

The many cardiac spouses who trusted me with their stories, their pain, their indomitable strength, and their recovery

The staff at Heartworks™—Dan Carey, Cathy Killeen, and Lori Pinkus—for their encouragement and staunch support of my work

Psychosynthesis, its principles and practitioners—it was within that framework that I opened to my sense of purpose

The mentors I've been privileged to learn from, especially Rene Schwartz, who gave me her wisdom and love, as I searched for my truth

Elizabeth Kübler-Ross, for her courage to cut a professional path that I could walk on and expand from

Ellen Sue Stern, who helped me transform my vision into a physical and accessible reality

Gareth Esersky, my editor at Prentice Hall Press, for believing in the book and giving to it her gifts of clarity and precision

My friends who have supported me as a cardiac spouse, and as a woman: Bonnie Barland, Shirley Kaplan, Vonnie Kilkelly, Eileen Rotman, Chelle Stillman, Harriet Swartz, and Sandy Swirnoff

My children, Sid and Debbie, who not always willingly shared my energy with the priority of this work, for their love

CONTENTS

Preface to the 1994 Edition

*I*t has been seven years since the publication of *Heart-mates® A Survival Guide for the Cardiac Spouse.* Heart disease continues unabated, and is our largest disabler and killer. Recent technological advances and pharmaceutical miracles have increased survival rates substantially. Although heartmates® has yet to become a household word, there may now be as many as twenty million of us.

The printing of this beautiful new edition gives me the opportunity to look back over these seven years to appreciate and recount progress, and to clarify what still needs to be accomplished.

Healthcare professionals at every level have embraced concepts outlined in the Heartmates® resources: coming to understand that when someone is given a cardiac diagnosis, goes through a procedure, or has a heart attack, the event involves more than the heart patient. The patient is a part of a larger unit, the family system, and the lives of all family members are changed forever by a cardiac event. As healthcare professionals expand the definition of who the patient is, they are beginning to treat the whole cardiac family.

A new field of study, dealing with the "vicarious victims of trauma," legitimizes the issues and needs of cardiac families experiencing a shocking and unexpected cardiac event.

Cardiac rehabilitation today includes Heartmates® principles and practices as a normal component of established programs. Many cardiac professionals report great satisfaction assisting cardiac spouses with their unique and universal needs. Nurses, social workers, and chaplains have welcomed the resource of the book, utilizing it as the foundation of cardiac spouse educational programs in hospitals and clinics.

Heartmates® is now available in French and German, and we are working on requests for Spanish and Hebrew editions.

I have been privileged to travel throughout the United States, Canada, and Israel training cardiac professionals and addressing cardiac couples. I have heard remarkable stories from and about the challenges cardiac families have encountered and triumphed over. Many newspaper and journal articles as well as radio and television interviews have clarified the crisis cardiac families face.

Understanding that family support and emotional factors play a significant role in the heart patient's as well as the cardiac family's recovery, Marion Laboratories commissioned me to create a series of educational videotapes for cardiac spouses and families to view in-hospital. These video programs, given to 5,000 hospitals as a public service in 1989-1990, have provided widespread recognition of the serious crisis sustained by cardiac families, and are designed to ease the heartmate's road to recovery.

Canada, with full support by Nordic Laboratories (a subsidiary of Marion Merrell Dow Inc.), has adopted all the Heartmates® resources for its cardiac families. Every clinic and hospital across Canada has the video programs in French or in English. Nordic Laboratories has also given hospitals my two hundred page professional manual, *The Cardiac Family Recovery Program Training Manual*, so that hospitals are prepared to provide appropriate programs and classes for their cardiac families.

Without Nordic and Marion Laboratories' support, literally hundreds of thousands of cardiac families would still be isolated and unprepared. Instead, because of their commitment, families are learning to accept heart disease as a part of their reality. They are able to emerge from the shock, and begin to live life anew, many experiencing new skills and understanding.

One of the most gratifying of my personal experiences has been that many, many heartmates® have written to me - - appreciating the book or the video programs, and expressing that they feel more understood and less alone. They have let me know specifically what has been of practical help, and what has given their spirits a needed boost. Each letter helps me to remain focused - - they remind me of the importance of continuing to work to bring the heartmate vision to fruition: that heartmates® everywhere will be recognized and supported, as we go about the tasks of healing our wounds, adjusting to our new family reality, and rebuilding our heartmate relationship.

I hope this book will help *you* with the experience of being a heartmate in recovery. Celebrate each milestone and give yourself permission to find joy in each precious day.

Rhoda Levin

Rhoda F. Levin

Minneapolis
March 1994

Foreword

*F*antasies and nightmares produce more unresolved fear than reality. Reality, faced in isolation, can be a nightmare. The reality of a heart attack is unclear because of the way it distorts and fragments the living patterns of a family. Even when the medical staff members suggest that it is a mild heart attack, the family must deal with the distress of unanswered and unanswerable questions. What is the likelihood of death? What will be the extent of disability? Fragments of information from diverse sources cause confusion and despair.

Ms. Levin's useful book, written for those with a spouse who has experienced a cardiac event, will be of great consolation to many. It is a guide to living as a tourist in the harsh, overpowering world of the hospital. It will be as close a companion as any tour book. It is a guide for providing home care for patients recovering from cardiac disease. It is a guide to the perplexing inner emotional experience of living through a heart attack with a spouse. Finally, it is a guide to the intimate handling of that most delicate of heart patients, the marriage.

Heartmates® brings help on many levels simultaneously. First and foremost, it is a handbook offering guidance for help in dealing with the hospital and medical staff, with feelings, the family, and marital intimacy. It offers suggestions for diet, coping with life-style changes, and it lists resource centers where information is available. There are many brief case examples from the experiences of other cardiac spouses. Finally, interwoven with wonderful delicacy, is the story of the author's experience with her husband's two heart attacks and successful bypass surgery. These personal samples are used to illustrate what is too ambiguous to describe. They appear in my memory of the book as trail markers on forest trees.

While the bright light of technological advance in medicine illuminates disease processes, improves survival rates, and reduces the disabling components of serious illness such as coronary artery disease, the human despair at the center of the experience remains hidden in darkness. The families of heart patients are subject to massive, long-term, often unacknowledged distress. The process leaves the family brittle and lacking resilience.

Case example: Several years ago the Swenson family was referred to me because Bill, age thirteen, the second of five children, had been arrested for vandalizing cars in their upper-middle-class neighborhood. It was not until the third family therapy interview that we discovered that the father, age forty-eight, had a coronary one year previously. It was no accident we were not told, because the family was under the father's strict orders not to speak of his heart attack. In his words, it had been a "mild" heart attack and "could have no possible effect" on the family. Over his protestations, his wife and children described their concern about their husband and father. They were angry that he remained seriously overweight and continued his heavy smoking. The mother said she had not had a full night's sleep since his heart attack, and every time he became upset with the children's fighting, she was fearful it would precipitate another attack. The father was very upset with me for encouraging his family to talk about their experiences. "It has nothing to do with my son's problems," he repeated emphatically. Yet the family's relief at being able to talk openly was obvious. The tough, taciturn thirteen-year-old vandal told freely about his fears that his father might die. Mr. Swenson refused to bring his family back for another interview. Six months later, the family doctor who had referred them told me that Bill had become a starter on the hockey team, and was back on the honor roll.

This case review gives an example of some less obvious side effects of coronary artery disease. *Heartmates®*

would have been invaluable to Mrs. Swenson in providing a support for her reality, which was at odds with her husband's. Her reality included her own anxiety symptoms, the distress she could see in their children, and her fantasies about what would happen if he died. His reality included only his doctor's suggestion that it was a mild heart attack and that he could resume his normal work schedule. He had no idea what his wife and children were experiencing and his denial of death was ludicrous.

Coronary artery disease can be a catastrophic and/or chronic illness, causing problems for the whole family. Health, both physical and psychological, is a function of a family's morale, the family's heart. The clinical tools for helping families under stress have evolved in the mental health professions, but have not been integrated into the medical world. Books like this one will educate the families of patients so that they can be more aware of the implications that serious illness in a family member has for them. As families come to understand the way they are affected by illness, it may lead to changes in the way medical practitioners view the experience of illness. If illness is placed in the context of family living patterns rather than in the simpler individual context, then families can be treated so that patterns of family living do not have a detrimental effect on a member who is ill. Instead, the patterns of family living can be guided so as to enhance recovery both for the patient and family.

— David V. Keith, M.D.
Director of Family Therapy
Associate Professor in Psychiatry
State University of New York
Health Science Center
Syracuse, New York

Introduction

As the spouse of someone who has survived the sudden onset of heart disease, you are in a special category, one that is relatively new in our society. In the last fifteen years, advanced medical technology and pharmaceutical discoveries have revolutionized the treatment of heart disease. Hardly a day goes by that we don't hear of a new study clarifying risk factors or announcing another technological breakthrough. Five hundred bypass surgeries and as many angioplasty procedures are done in our country every day. Billions of dollars are spent on medical treatment and research. The predicted number of heart attacks annually in the United States is 1.5 million. Of these, *more than 1 million will survive.* Each year the number of cardiac spouses grows. Today there may be as many as 20 million of us.

Strange as it seems, it may be easier in some ways to be widowed than to be the spouse of a recovering heart patient. There are role models for widows' behavior, and appropriate ways to express difficult emotions. People respect the time it takes for the widowed to adjust to the changes in their lives.

Cardiac spouses have no role models, teachers, or mentors. No one, professional or friend, can tell you what specific changes you will face as a cardiac spouse, and yet *change is your reality.*

When my husband had his first heart attack, I felt totally unprepared. I was forty-three, an urban mother, wife

1

of an architect, and well established in my second professional career.

Marsh and I were typical 1950s high-school sweethearts. He was the football hero and I the adoring coed. The future looked unlimited from where we stood. We were both bright and talented. College provided us with an additional layer of confidence, optimism, and idealism. I felt like Wonder Woman: healthy, invincible, and protected by her magic bracelets. It never dawned on me that I was marrying anyone less than Superman.

Our first adventure in the early 1960s was to leave the safety of Minneapolis and make our way in the Big Apple. Marsh, a Coast Guard officer, was stationed in the battery in New York City. I taught English in an all-black junior high school in a well-to-do New Jersey suburb. We involved ourselves in the desegregation movement: Marsh through sports and I through my work with adolescents. It was exciting and satisfying to come out of those years believing that our lives were meaningful. We were committed to living them as an adventure and making the world a better place. I felt that if we just worked hard and believed in justice we could do anything. I had felt neither danger nor limitation.

In 1966, Marsh's Dad died of a heart attack. Three months later, we left for Tunis, Tunisia, to serve in the Peace Corps. We were of the generation that could respond to John F. Kennedy's call to serve: a little too old to be flower children and still too young for his assassination to suggest danger or mortality for ourselves. Getting by the dangers, real or imagined, of being Jewish in an Arab country during the Six-day War, and of being pregnant and having our first baby two continents away from home and family, added to my sense of invincibility. We were strong and resilient, and we returned to Minneapolis in 1968 unscathed and triumphant.

During our early thirties, our adventures were focused within our individual professional fields. Marsh's energy went toward his work in architecture. I went back to school to earn a graduate degree in social work. We had a second child, and struggled somewhat separately and silently with the problems of keeping careers and family intact. My mother died when I was thirty-five, and that experience taught me that I was vulnerable. If my mother could die, then I could too. But death and illness still seemed very far away. I never considered at that time that Marsh could die.

Approaching our forties, having achieved success in our careers, our restlessness and our search for meaning were renewed. Marsh tried a career change; my idealism uprooted us again, and with our two little ones, we left Minneapolis for San Francisco to work within the human potential movement.

By the fall of 1980, I was ready to return home. We hadn't changed the world; we saw a lot more violence and danger than ever before. We were disappointed and disillusioned. Wounded by the reality, but still believing in *our* resilience and invincibility, we started over again.

Our expectations of what we could and should accomplish were scaled down; we were maturing. We were concerned about rebuilding a safe and secure home back in Minneapolis for our family. Marsh returned to architecture; we bought a house and I began to rebuild my therapy practice. On the night of November 16, 1981, as we lay in bed watching "Monday Night Football," Marsh turned to me and said, "Don't get scared, but I think I'm having a heart attack." That moment was the last of my old life, a life in which I had thought we would live and triumph over everything and every situation, forever. It was also the first moment of my *new* life, a life that included being a cardiac spouse.

Marsh *was* having a heart attack that night. Nine weeks later he had a second heart attack. Luckily, both left him with minimal heart damage. Regaining his strength,

Marsh returned to work full time and to a life with few physical restrictions. He went faithfully to a cardiac rehabilitation class three times a week, which also functioned as an emotional support group for him.

I recovered from the shock of becoming a cardiac spouse at age forty-three, but I was more confused than ever before in my life. Every aspect of my life was in flux: All my old beliefs had failed me; my security was lost; even my daily life-style was different. Marsh wasn't invincible and neither was I. My feeling of being in control of the life and well-being of our family had vanished. My experience as a clinical social worker helped me identify that I was in crisis. But wherever I turned, I felt alone. I couldn't find a support group to attend. There wasn't one book available that spoke to the issues I was facing.

I stumbled around, trying to deal with the uncertainty and the real changes, and after a year and a half decided to start a program that could help me and other cardiac spouses. Ironically, I was scheduled to present my program to a local hospital's cardiac rehabilitation team that very week in the late fall of 1983 when Marsh's plateau ended. He was scheduled for an angiogram on Wednesday; I presented the Heartmates® program on Thursday; and Marsh had quadruple bypass surgery on Friday. Recovery for each of us and for our relationship took longer psychologically than physically. It was disappointing and difficult to have to start over again.

I have written this book because I believe recovery is possible, for me and for you. In this book I share what I've learned from my own experience and from the opportunity to work with many cardiac spouses in the Heartmates® program. My hope is that you will identify with, and be strengthened by reading about, others who struggle with issues similar to your own.

My intention has been to write for all cardiac spouses, men and women alike. At the present time, only a small percentage of cardiac spouses are male, but their numbers continue to rise. In relation to my use of language, I have chosen to subordinate semantics to my message. After considering the use of he/she, I chose to use the traditional he, trusting that no one will be alienated or offended.

There has been up to now a lack of recognition about the emotional dimension of the cardiac crisis and heart disease. It is my hope that cardiologists, thoracic surgeons, and cardiac nurses will read *Heartmates®* and will continue the progress already begun to close the gap between physical medicine and caring for the whole person, as well as the family system. I wish for all of us that competent and compassionate care becomes the standard for patients, their spouses, and families.

Full recovery depends on a balance between the healing of the physical being and the psyche. For that reason, this book combines and interweaves practical information, psychological support, and emotional guidance.

Each cardiac spouse is unique, and every cardiac situation is different. This book does not propose a specific cure for living with the realities of heart disease. It does include suggestions, tips, and tools. What works for one person or couple may not be effective for others. Consider all specific suggestions as ideas with which to experiment, suggestions to be molded to fit your own personal needs and situation.

The book is arranged chronologically, beginning in the hospital and moving through aspects of recovery. But because of the ongoing nature of heart disease, the setbacks and plateaus that complicate recovery, you may want to reread the early chapters often, even if you are a longtime veteran.

At another level, the book goes from the elementary to the complex, from the simple and more obvious changes to deeper issues and questions. Themes in later chapters are recovery and the healing of relationships with your mate, your family, and yourself. These issues are fundamental to the ultimate quality of our lives, but for most of us, they are the last to be recognized and dealt with.

The challenge of the cardiac crisis is facing the reality of your situation, letting go of what is lost, and developing new ways to live that enhance the quality of your life. My experience has deepened my belief that *relationships are what matter most.* I have strengthened my commitment to myself and to my marriage. I try to appreciate each day as it comes and cherish the precious gifts of life and love.

I hope that you will rely on this book as you journey through your cardiac crisis. *Heartmates*® is meant to be such a guide. It is also a reminder that you are not alone. Accept my support and the shared experience of the many others in this book who reach out to stand with you as well, as you deal with the difficulties and opportunities of being a heartmate.

At the Hospital

*M*y heart racing, I park and run through the darkness toward the double doors marked Emergency. Where is my husband? The ambulance he arrived in stands empty and there is no sign of him. Only an hour ago we were safely curled up in bed, watching TV and comparing notes on the details of our day. His sudden chest pain and an urgent call to 911 have led me to this door, where I stop, take a deep breath, and realize I don't know what to do.

Once inside, I am jolted by the glare of artificial light, medicinal smells, and an operator's strident voice repeatedly paging doctors. I need to get my bearings, gather my composure, and figure out a plan. But I'm frantic, not knowing whether Marsh has had a heart attack or is even alive.

I approach the registration desk and I am directed to Admitting. A woman behind a computer says to be seated, she will call me. The minutes tick by. I try to keep from screaming at her to hurry up. Doesn't she know this is an emergency? Finally she begins the ritual list of questions establishing identity, financial responsibility, and the nature of the complaint. I search my mind for Marsh's social security number and my wallet for insurance information. I can't believe I'm wasting time doing this when I should be with Marsh. When she's finished, I'm motioned back to the waiting room to resume my vigil.

7

After an hour, I am told that Marsh is being taken to Coronary Care. I ride with him on the elevator, but when we reach the fifth floor I'm waved away to wait in the family lounge. I'm not sure what's happening. It seems certain that Marsh has had a heart attack, but how sick is he? When can I see him? Where is the doctor? Should I stay all night or go home to be with our children and try to get some sleep? How can I possibly sleep? If I leave, will he die?

My body is numb. My mind races a million miles an hour with questions coming so fast and furiously that one begins where the last one leaves off. I'm tempted to escape this nightmare but I don't know how. Instead, I brace myself and walk into the coronary unit. Rules are posted at the nurses' station. Visitors are allowed ten minutes each hour, only one person at a time. My eyes are riveted by a half dozen monitors, each silently recording ongoing lines that are images of the patients' heart-beats. On one, the green line is zigzagging uncontrollably in an ominous pattern. What if it's Marsh's? What should I do? I tell myself to take it easy; I don't even know how the machine works.

The nurse calmly informs me that Marsh is resting comfortably and that I can see him for just a few minutes. Everything is quiet and controlled here, the sounds absorbed by carpeting. I imitate the nurse's measured tone, lowering my voice before entering Marsh's room.

Now, after two excruciating hours, I stand at Marsh's bedside. I don't know what to say. Marsh is all wired up. There's an oxygen tube in his nose and an intravenous line dripping liquid into his wrist. He is attached to a machine that gives a digital readout of his pulse; it is equipped with a miniature version of the screen at the nurse's desk. Again I stare at the critical green line that mysteriously makes its way from left to right, reappearing again and again.

Marsh says he knows he has had a heart attack, but that he isn't in any pain. He asks me to take care of some arrangements at the office and jokes about canceling his breakfast date since he obviously won't be there. His ashen skin and frightened eyes belie his businesslike manner and his humor. I'm not sure how to act and whether or not to show how worried I am. Before I've had a chance to sort out my feelings, the nurse signals that my time is up. I lean over to kiss Marsh, careful not to disturb the lifesaving equipment.

On my way out, I stop at the desk for reassurance that Marsh will be okay if I leave. The nurse says it's fine to call

any time, day or night. I find my car in the lot and drive home,
where I collapse into our bed and sleep fitfully until dawn.

Whether your introduction to being a cardiac spouse started with your mate's heart attack or bypass surgery, your crisis began as all do, suddenly and without warning. While heart disease develops over a long period of time, a cardiac crisis happens in an instant. You might have noticed gradual signs, such as your spouse's shortness of breath, or pallor that is unlike his familiar ruddy complexion. But nothing prepared you for the terrifying split-second when you witnessed his heart attack. Nor for the seemingly routine checkup that indicated the immediate need for an angiogram, angioplasty, or bypass surgery. At that moment, you were catapulted into a new and frightening reality. With no time to absorb what had happened and no way to know what was ahead, you were propelled into action and forced to deal with a life-and-death crisis.

In many ways, a cardiac crisis is similar to other life-threatening emergencies. However, cardiac spouses share the unique experience of being in a crisis precipitated by someone else's illness. Your mate is in crisis too, but the experience is not the same. You suddenly find yourself in a situation entirely beyond your control that threatens your security and will change your future. Unless you have medical training, you are faced with a foreign vocabulary of medical terms you can barely pronounce, let alone understand.[1] You may have to decipher this technical information in order to make decisions with far-reaching consequences on behalf of your mate. And to top it all off, the one person on whom you rely is totally unavailable. Instead of operating as part of a team, you must deal with this all on your own.

In a crisis, the initial reaction is often numbness. Cardiac spouses describe a sense of being removed from reality, as if they are walking around in a dense fog. During the first few days, you may have trouble concentrating, making decisions, and carrying on conversations with relatives and friends. These are typical reactions. The body shuts down in response to shock to prevent being overwhelmed. It serves as a protective shield, masking the intensity of feelings, allowing you to continue functioning. This is usually a temporary reaction which quickly passes. At this time it's wise to preserve your energy, and handle only those tasks and decisions that absolutely cannot wait.

Living in Limbo

Once the numbness wears off, you will probably become fearful. The most compelling fear is that your spouse won't survive. Despite medical evidence to the contrary, it is natural to associate a heart attack with death. And even though bypass surgery has an impressive track record, it inevitably evokes fear and anxiety.

Anxiety, often as not, manifests itself physically. During the first days, while you wait for conclusive information about your husband's condition, you may feel like a tightly wound spring, ready to snap at the slightest provocation. Other symptoms include loss of appetite, trembling, shallow breathing, or insomnia. One spouse noticed her arm ached and realized she had been constantly clenching her fist. Another developed a nervous habit of biting her lip. Fear paralyzes some people, makes others withdrawn, and causes still others to become overactive, aimlessly pacing the corridors of the hospital or chattering incessantly.

The hours spent waiting during surgery can be the most difficult of all. While it may help to have close friends and family around for distraction and support, ultimately you are alone with your fears. Thoughts about the outcome of surgery bring up a set of survival questions that keep you holding your breath. Will he be in that small percentage that doesn't make it through bypass surgery? Will his heart beat on its own after being connected to the heart-lung machine? Will he breathe when they remove the respirator? Will he get pneumonia? How long will the new arteries work, or will they just collapse? There's no way to speed up time, and the surgeon's words, "The surgery was successful; all vital signs are stable," are only a partial remedy.

Seeing Marsh lying in the intensive care unit was dramatically different from anything I could have imagined. There were neither windows nor clocks in the cubicle and time felt indefinitely suspended. Marsh's hold on life seemed very tenuous. Every part of him was hooked up to something. He was at the center of a whirlwind of activity. Skilled, efficient nurses moved swiftly in and out, executing complex life-sustaining procedures. I knew that morphine protected Marsh from pain, but he was restless and straining against the respirator. His hand and arm, still chilled from surgery, felt like a stranger's. All the while the regular rhythm of the monitors reassured me with their beep. . .beep. . .beep. I returned to the waiting room totally shaken by what I had seen. Marsh couldn't even breathe on his own. How would he ever be healthy and whole again?

Once the initial crisis passes, your worries continue, intensified by the unknown nature of heart disease. While you are relieved that your mate has survived, new questions arise. What are the details of his condition, and what is the long-term prognosis? Will your spouse have constant pain? Will he be dependent on medication? Is he going to be an invalid? Will he be able to work, to travel, to lead an active and fulfilling life? What are the chances of another heart attack?

Most of us have a hard time coping with the unknown. Learning to live with uncertainty is one of the greatest challenges for the partner of someone with heart disease. Knowing that your mate is in competent professional hands can alleviate fear. While it's essential to get all the information and medical guidance you need, it's also important to recognize that even the most gifted physicians cannot foretell the future. The best they can provide are percentages for recovery. Medicine, for all its awesome accomplishments, is still a limited science.

Your anxiety will diminish as you become more secure about your mate's survival and as the repercussions of his illness become clear. In the meantime, voice your concerns. In some hospitals, trained social workers and chaplains are available to help you through this traumatic time. Acknowledging your fear to someone or to yourself can reduce its power, as shown in the following story.

Ruth, a soft-spoken woman in her early fifties, drove her husband forty miles to the hospital emergency room. After his examination, she was told to follow him and his entourage of medical staff to the intensive care unit. At the big double doors she was stopped and told to wait outside. No one explained what was happening. Ruth sat alone in the silent corridor for close to an hour. During that time she considered every possibility. She didn't think she would ever see Ralph alive again. She reviewed the highlights of their thirty years together, thinking about what he meant to her and how much she would miss him. She recalled their dreams and tried to imagine pursuing them alone. She even planned his funeral, picturing herself there with their three sons.

The doors of the intensive care unit swung open and a nurse emerged. Ruth, lost in her own thoughts, was startled. The nurse told her that Ralph was doing well and all vital signs were stable. She burst into tears of joy and relief. But the hour Ruth had spent waiting was a turning point in her life. She had prepared herself emotionally for the loss of her husband and confronted squarely the idea of living as a widow. Ruth rose to go to her husband feeling strengthened and confident in her ability to cope with this new reality.

In the midst of crisis, fears intensify and get blown

out of proportion. The urgency of the situation makes it almost impossible to keep things in perspective. Lack of information increases dread and permits you to imagine worst-case scenarios. We are so accustomed to having physicians provide clear answers that any vagueness or gray area can be interpreted as bad news. Some people naturally cope with the unknown by adopting a positive attitude—they know survival is a given. Others are more likely to envision the worst. When told that 98 percent of the people who have bypass surgery survive, they automatically place themselves with the remaining 2 percent.

Anxiety in the face of the unknown is a normal and appropriate response, as long as it doesn't impair your ability to function. Go ahead with a cautious optimism — the combination of a positive outlook with a realistic appreciation for the gravity of the situation. That way you can hope for the best and still be prepared to cope with any contingencies.

Making Yourself at Home

As you struggle with your fear about your mate's survival and recovery, you need to deal simultaneously with a new and strange environment. Trading the familiarity of home for the alien atmosphere of the hospital further distorts your reality and gives you the feeling of disorientation. Your schedule is completely out of kilter, and your sense of time is governed by hospital routine: rotating shifts, the return of the latest test results, and the doctor's rounds. For all intents and purposes, you have taken up residence at the hospital. You may spend periods of time at work or at home, but your mind and your heart are somewhere else.

How do you handle the hospital? First, you must recognize what part the hospital plays in your emotional experience. On one hand, it's a relief to see your spouse safely ensconced, attended by professionals who can prolong, and, in some instances, save his life. On the other hand, the hospital system is not designed with your needs in mind. The physical layout, regimented pace, and antiseptic environment is geared toward maximum care and increased productivity. Its primary purpose is to accommodate the patients and medical staff.

It goes without saying that your first priority is your mate's recovery. However, you too have needs, basic human needs that arise in a crisis, including: the need to belong, the need to be needed, the need for information, and the need for support. In order to feel comfortable, you must first understand the lay of the land. Find your way around, know the location of the lounge, the telephone, the gift shop, the coffee shop, and the chapel—doing so will contribute to a semblance of order. It's frustrating to find yourself on the Employee Only elevator en route to the supply room, missing a long-awaited ten-minute visit with your mate. And the fact that most family lounges are hidden away in an obscure corner adds nothing to your feelings of connection and belonging.

Once you get your bearings, the next step is to understand the inner workings of the system. This is what I call "cracking the code." A hospital is a unique world, with its own language, customs, and culture. Your aim is to effectively maneuver and negotiate on behalf of yourself and your spouse. This necessitates learning the procedures, vocabulary, and chain of command.

At times you may feel frustrated or in the way. Everyone else rushes around doing an important job, while you hurry up and wait: for visiting hours, for fifteen minutes with the doctor, for test results, for rehabilitation meetings. In some ways your needs seem at cross-purposes with the running of the hospital. You trust your cardiologist's competence more when you see how busy he is. But because of

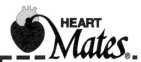

Heartmates® resources are designed to serve the cardiac spouse and family during and after a cardiac crisis. Future educational materials may be available to help cardiac families. To be included on our mailing list, please print your name and address below. Thank you for answering these questions to assist in future research by Heartmates®. My personal best for a full recovery to both of you. *Rhoda Hevi*

Patient's age:_____ Male ☑ Female ☑
   Your age:_____ Male ☑ Female ☑
Date of most recent cardiac event: _____
What heart medication, if any, has been prescribed?
_____

Specifically, how was the book, *Heartmates®* useful to you?
_____
_____

What has changed most in your life since the onset of your mate's heart disease?_____
_____

Please check (X) any of the following topics that you are concerned about or are interested in:

_____ Finances	_____ Work
_____ Depression	_____ Fear/Anxiety
_____ Lifestyle Changes	_____ Travel
_____ Physical Intimacy	_____ Smoking
_____ Grief	_____ Family/Children
_____ Anger/Irritability	_____ Communication

Other: _____

Indicate your preferred format:
☐ Videotape   ☐ Audiotape   ☐ Printed Materials

NAME _____
ADDRESS _____
CITY_____ PROV. _____
POSTAL ZONE _____ PHONE (____)_____

Heartmates® Inc
c/o TTS Distributing, Inc.
45 Tyler Street
P.O. Box 425
Aurora, ON L4G 9Z9

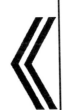

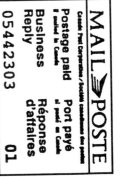

his pressing schedule, he makes his rounds before you can get there in the morning or in the only half hour you leave to get a cup of coffee. And when you finally catch up with him, you have forgotten the one question you meant to ask. You admire the nurses' ability to handle so many things at once. But the fact that they're so busy makes you hesitant to bother them with your questions. After a while, it all starts to seem like a conspiracy to keep you in the dark.

There is nothing you can do to change the nursing staff's style, but you have every right to ask them questions. If there never seems to be an appropriate time to do so, set up a specific time to discuss your concerns. It's unlikely that you are going to change your doctor's schedule. But you might try calling his office to find out when he will be on hospital premises or make a formal appointment instead of anxiously waiting for his appearance.

Cardiac spouses often perceive the hospital staff as a lifeline, but this can make you feel very dependent on them. Such dependence can, in turn, cause you to be especially careful in your relationships with the nurses and doctors. You may worry about asking too many questions or being labeled pushy or demanding. You might be afraid of making a wrong move, inadvertently doing something to antagonize the nurses and jeopardize your mate's care.

Whether or not it's justified, it doesn't take long to get the idea that if you're "good" and wait patiently without making waves, your mate will benefit from first-class service by the staff. One cardiac spouse never came to the hospital without bringing candy for the nurses. Another always prefaced her questions with an apology, fearing the nurses would think she was stupid or wasting their time.

Many cardiac spouses are reluctant to express their opinions, thinking that their input will be construed as interference or doubt.

Early in Marsh's hospitalization, I wrestled with the

conflict between my desire to be seen as a "cooperative spouse" and my need to participate in his care. In an educational session with the coronary care nurse, Marsh and I were shown a chart of "mets," the units of energy expended in each physical activity. It covered the period from the heart attack through six weeks of recovery, listing the graduated activities that would ultimately lead to resuming a normal life.

The following day, Marsh was moved to a cardiac recovery unit. A nurse appeared and informed him that he had bathroom privileges. I knew she was wrong. According to the "mets" chart, bathroom privileges were several days off. Although it wasn't ten yards away, I reacted as if Marsh was being encouraged to sprint around a track or take an extra base on an infield single. As much as I wanted him back on his feet, part of me wished he could permanently remain in coronary care and never again do anything that took any "mets" at all. Why tempt fate? Better he should do nothing more active than breathe, love me, and live.

I didn't want the stigma of "trouble," but I was determined that Marsh not get out of bed until the chart permitted. I found the charge nurse, waited until she was free, and told her that Marsh did not have bathroom privileges and wouldn't for several days. Once I said this, my fear subsided. In its place a new dread appeared: if this mistake could be made, I'd better stay watchful and alert in case a bigger or more dangerous one occurred. If it were necessary, I'd move in and stand guard twenty-four hours a day.

Combatting Helplessness

It's natural to feel helpless when you are caught up in events beyond your control. In some ways you are truly helpless. Nothing you can do will turn back the clock. You can neither change nor ignore the fact that your spouse has heart disease. There's no way to reverse the risk factors and life-style choices that contributed to this crisis. And unless you are medically trained you are incapable of providing the technical care that's required. It's important to acknowledge these realities, but it's equally valuable to recognize your power.

Most of us endow physicians with too much power. In a crisis we're apt to expect physicians to work miracles. Terrified, we expect them to have all the answers and never make mistakes. Once we make the doctors omnipotent, it's difficult to have appropriate expectations of them. And by giving up so much power to your doctor, you diminish your own. If you have a question or idea, you may stifle it, thinking, "I've never been to medical school," or "If the doctor thought it was necessary, he'd have recommended it." What you don't take into account is that no physician knows everything. Regardless of how smart or dedicated a doctor is, no one can keep up with every new development in a field. Your doctor is the medical expert, but you know more about your mate than anyone else does. And no one cares as much as you and your husband about his full recovery. Sharing your knowledge can be crucial in planning his recovery program with the staff.

You can increase your power by educating yourself about heart disease. The more you know, the more you will be able to contribute to your spouse's recovery. Christina, an avid reader, came across a ten-year study of a medication thought to reduce cholesterol rates. A year earlier, her husband, Paul, had undergone bypass surgery and she wondered if the newly available medication might be a significant addition to his exercise and diet program of recovery. Christina clipped the article and showed it to their doctor, who followed up and prescribed the medication.

Sometimes we withhold valuable information because we feel intimidated or shy. But your intimate relationship with your spouse makes it especially important for you to speak up. Stuart, a quiet and intuitive man, felt terribly uneasy sitting beside his dozing wife, Kim, the first night following her bypass surgery. Despite assurances that Kim was in stable condition, he was seized with an irrational sense of foreboding. Something was wrong, and while he couldn't put his finger on it, the feeling was impossible to dismiss. When a nurse passed, Stuart asked her to check Kim, who indeed was developing post surgical complications. Within minutes, emergency measures were taken and a potential disaster prevented.

Information is another factor in counteracting helplessness. It is your need, your right, and your responsibility to have access to all the available data.

Under state law, we are protected by a "Patients' Bill of Rights." (Ask for a copy of your bill of rights from your nurse or hospital social worker.) Among twenty-six sections of the Minnesota bill are four that are especially pertinent to cardiac family members:

1. Patients have the right to be treated by the staff with courtesy and respect for their individuality.
2. Patients have the right to be given complete and current information concerning their diagnoses, treatment alternatives, risks, and prognoses, in language they can be expected to understand.
3. Patients (including a family member) have the right to participate in the planning of their health care.
4. Patients have the right to a prompt and reasonable response to their questions and requests.

HEARTMATES® HOSPITAL QUESTIONS

The following list is a guide for asking questions and gathering information. As you read over the items, note the questions that concern you the most, and add new ones as you go along.

Heart Attack
1. What is a heart attack?
2. What does heart damage mean?
3. How long does recovery take?
4. Will my spouse need open heart surgery?
5. What causes a heart attack?

Medications
1. What is the medication supposed to do?
2. What are the potential side effects?
3. How long will the drug need to be taken?
4. How frequently is it taken?
5. What happens if a dose is missed?
6. What is the generic name of the drug?
7. What are the reasons for changes in medications?
8. What should we do if he can't remember having taken his pills?

Surgery and Procedures
1. What is angioplasty? What is bypass surgery?
2. When is angioplasty or surgery indicated?
3. What are the advantages? The risks?
4. Who is best qualified to do the surgery?
5. Where can we get a second opinion?
6. How soon should the procedure or surgery be done?
7. How long does it take to recover from angioplasty? From bypass surgery?

Recovery
1. When will my mate be able to come home?
2. What life-style changes should be made?
3. Will he have to change his job or retire early?
4. What kind of emotional reactions should I expect from my spouse? How long will he be depressed or angry?

5. Will we be able to resume sexual activity? When?
   Are there any dangers involved in having intercourse?
6. How often should we schedule appointments with
   the doctor? Will the hospital provide any ongoing
   support? Whom should I call to answer my questions?

Your list of questions is undoubtedly lengthy and
will change daily. Put them in writing to help remember
them, and to mark the significance of your concerns and
bolster your confidence. Once you have compiled a list,
decide who can best respond. Some questions should be
directed to your cardiologist. Others require the expertise
of the nursing staff, the exercise physiologist, the nutrition-
ist, or a veteran cardiac spouse.

You are absolutely entitled to all the information
you need. If the answers you receive are too vague, like,
"Oh, that's nothing to worry about" (easy for you to say), or
"Time will take care of that" (how much time?), be prepared
to ask again. In some instances, an unsatisfactory answer
may be precipitated by an unclear question. You may need
to be more specific. In other cases communication problems are more complex.

Some doctors are comfortable answering questions
and are sensitive to your feelings and concerns. Others are
defensive, unresponsive, and noncommittal. They may
brush off your questions for a number of reasons, including
time pressures, lack of communication skills, and discomfort discussing issues that are painful or ambiguous.

Ideally, your doctor is someone whose medical
knowledge you trust and with whom you are personally
comfortable. More likely, as in any relationship, there are
compromises. Your doctor may be a respected expert in
cardiology, but he may have limited experience in a variety
of surgical procedures. He may enjoy the best medical
reputation in town, while his bedside manner may leave
something to be desired.

What matters is knowing what will make you feel most secure. Out of loyalty to your doctor, you may feel that you should unconditionally accept his judgments. In truth, your only obligation is to pursue a course of treatment that will facilitate your mate's recovery and your peace of mind. If you're unsure after his diagnosis, seek a second opinion. If the two conflict, get a third. If you and your mate are ill at ease with your doctor, look for another.

Bridging Communication

Assertive action enables you to be useful in another way. When someone you love is hurting, it's normal to want to help. During the hospital stay your contribution seems superfluous; from the moment your mate arrives, professionals and technology take over and you are relegated to the background. You would do anything in the world to help, but it feels like there's nothing to do.

Actually, there are many ways to be of use. There are at least two ways in which you can act as a bridge immediately following surgery: by acting as an intermediary between your mate and the busy professional staff, and as a connection to reality for your mate.

Right after surgery your spouse is totally vulnerable. The presence of a respirator and throat tubes make even verbal communication impossible. He has no way to make his simplest needs known. One practical suggestion is to use a "magic slate" (the children's toy) to help your husband express what he wants. There are things you can do for him yourself. Moistening dry lips, moving a sheet that's pulling on a tube, or readjusting a pillow can be important for both of you. Other things may require the expertise of the nurse. Your spouse may be anxious about a machine that has changed the rhythm of its "beep," and you can ask the nurse to explain.

Checking on medications is another way to act like a bridge. You can actively participate in your mate's care by becoming familiar with the name, dosage, and purposes of drugs being administered. Your spouse will feel some control over his own care if he can monitor his medications for dosage accuracy and take them on time. Both of you will feel more secure if you understand how the medications work.

The first few days following surgery are distinguished by a drug-induced "haze" which protects your spouse from pain, but may also cause him alternately to doze, be easily startled, be out of touch with reality, or say bizarre things. One woman reported that her husband thought he was being experimented on in a concentration camp. Another man admonished his family to hurry to the midnight buffet on the promenade deck of their cruise ship.

Your presence is significant to your mate because it is a symbol of stability and reality at a time of extreme confusion and vulnerability. With no other frame of reference available to him, you are your husband's connection to his earthly roots, his home, his family, his recovery, his life. Add powerful medication to an absence in the cardiac care unit of windows or clocks, and the already strange environment can be overwhelming. Simply telling the patient the time and whether it is day or night can provide him with an important reality check. Letting him know how long he's been there may furnish significant direction for his return to the world of life and the living.

Nourishing Yourself

Being a bridge is both a gift to your mate and a way to reduce your helplessness. By giving, you increase your power. But it's equally important to be able to receive. In a cardiac crisis, everyone's focus is understandably on the patient. However, you, too, are physically and emotionally vulnerable. Your daily schedule has been disrupted, you are spending most of your waking hours at the hospital, you are deeply affected by your mate's illness, and you are trying to juggle your spouse's needs with the other demands in your life.

Adequate rest and proper nutrition are two things that are often neglected in a crisis. This can lower your resistance and make you more susceptible to illness. You must eat regularly and get sufficient sleep. Hospital food is usually marginal, so it's a good idea to eat a nutritious breakfast at home. You might also pack a bag lunch and bring healthy snacks to eat in the family lounge. You need to keep your energy and spirits up, and, besides, a shared snack can be an ice-breaker in an otherwise tense situation.

Even if you are normally sedentary, take a walk at least once a day. Take a break from the confines of the hospital and get some fresh air. Just being in the outside world can replenish your resources.

I can't emphasize enough the importance of support. With the amount of pressure you are under, you run the risk of becoming depleted or resentful unless you nourish yourself too. This is an appropriate time to let yourself be taken care of by friends and relatives who are willing to bring food, accompany you on a walk, or visit with your spouse so that you can take a break. If ever you need and deserve support, it's now. There's no reason to try to do it all alone.

Before You Leave...

Many hospitals offer cardiac patients and spouses an educational program to provide information about diet, exercise, risk factors, stress, and sexuality. These classes are usually held while your mate is still hospitalized with the purpose of preparing you to go home.

In order to facilitate this process, let your nurses and doctors know what you need. It's safe to assume that the hospital staff members want to help, that their goal is to promote healing. That doesn't make them mind readers. Tell the staff if you have forgotten a detail from an earlier meeting and would appreciate hearing it again. If you are having trouble concentrating, say so. Be specific about areas that concern you, and keep on asking questions until you get the answers. If you feel embarrassed by your lack of knowledge, remember that you are in a totally new situation. These sessions are for you, so be sure to take advantage of the information and support.

Later, let the staff know how practical and worthwhile the educational sessions were. Your feedback is bound to benefit cardiac families in the future. And the staff, committed to quality care, will appreciate your perspective.

A good educational and support program will:

- Keep educational meetings short (no more than ten to fifteen minutes).
- Provide time for each couple to discuss the information with each other during each session.
- Make a question box available for individuals who are uncomfortable speaking in a group.
- Offer at least one meeting for cardiac spouses to identify their most pressing questions and concerns regarding preparations to take their spouses home.
- Provide clear and simple handouts covering the material discussed.

As you two move into the recovery phase, you may want to participate in an educational program that meets regularly. This can be very valuable as you make the transition from the acute crisis into the next stage, which brings its own new issues and concerns.

The hospital experience is only the beginning of a long-term situation heralded by the cardiac crisis. Issues that begin here will follow you home. You will have to learn to deal effectively with the medical community; it's just one part of life with someone who has a chronic condition. A positive way to approach this is to develop an ongoing relationship with your hospital staff members.

Since heart disease is incurable, this may not be your only time at the hospital. Nine weeks after Marsh's first heart attack, he had a second one. Two years later, sudden changes in his condition brought him back to the hospital for an angiogram followed by bypass surgery. Should you need to return to the hospital, you'll feel more at home if you have participated in educational programs and meetings in the interim.

In time, you will adjust more and more to living with uncertainty, but there will continue to be areas over which you have no control. You do not have the power to eradicate your spouse's heart disease or eliminate its effects on your life. Your primary goal, as you anticipate bringing your mate home from the hospital, is to be prepared to support his recovery and yours.

On the Road to Recovery

*T*he phone hasn't stopped ringing all morning. Everyone wants to know when Marsh will be home so they can come over to see him. Soon everything will be back to normal, and our lives will be just the same as they were before his heart attack. Driving to the hospital, I feel eager and excited. The days have seemed like forever. I'm grateful that there were no complications, that this nightmare is almost over.

I arrive in Marsh's room at the same time as his favorite nurse. Upbeat and professional, she carries a thick packet of papers which she ceremoniously turns over to me. In it are exercise diagrams and schedules, cholesterol tables, and scores of heart-healthy recipes. The nurse gives us a last reminder about avoiding undue stress and checks to make sure that Marsh has his medications for this afternoon. Finally, she hands me several prescriptions and instructs me to have them filled immediately.

I feel somewhat reassured by her orderliness and efficiency, but I'm a little nervous about taking Marsh home. I'm not sure if he's strong enough to wait in the car while I stop at the drugstore, or if I should drop him off at home and then go to fill the prescriptions. I don't know what to do, and my head is full of conflicting details and directions. I'm beginning to feel as though I've accepted a "Mission Impossible" assignment without fully realizing how difficult and dangerous it might be.

26

The nurse insists on pushing Marsh in a wheelchair. She assures me that he's fine, that it's hospital policy, but I feel like I'm taking home an invalid.

The back seat of the car is filled with gifts, books, and six large plants that Marsh accumulated during his stay. We're finally on our way home, the two of us, surrounded by symbols of life and love from all his well-wishers.

We stop at our neighborhood drugstore, and I rush in to get the pills. It seems to take forever to count out a few pills and label the bottles. The total comes to almost forty dollars. I'm shocked at the cost, but I quickly write a check and rush back to Marsh. He looks a little worn. I think about "undue stress" as I drive toward home and decide not to mention how expensive the prescriptions are.

Tears of joy fill my eyes as the kids throw their arms around Marsh to welcome him home. They stick around to keep us company while I unpack. I arrange the plants all around the bedroom because I want the "healing green" to be near Marsh. But it still looks like a sick room, with the hospital water pitcher, the medicine bottles, and the pile of new books.

By this time Marsh says he is tired and is going to take a nap. It's hard for me to imagine how he could be tired from just riding home from the hospital, but I say nothing and leave him to sleep.

I sit down with my packet of recipes and instructions, but I can't concentrate. I'm drained, but too wound up to relax. I feel disappointed that we haven't really talked or celebrated his homecoming. For days we have lived in public view, and I have had to share him with doctors, nurses, and technicians. The logical voice in my head begins to instruct me about what I should be thinking and feeling. "Calm down," it says. "You should lighten up, feel grateful, say a prayer of thanksgiving. Everything will be just like it used to be."

It wasn't. That first day home was only the beginning of the emotional upheaval that followed. Little did I know how much Marsh's heart attack had already changed my life.

What happened to me and *what is happening to you* is this: You have lived through the beginning phase of a crisis. You are beginning to adjust to changes that began abruptly and are beyond your control. These changes have already affected you, and will continue to have an impact on your life in ways that you cannot yet predict. Although you don't have heart disease, every part of you is vulnerable to the cardiac crisis.

The myth is that everything will be the same as it was. The truth is that *nothing will ever be the same again.*

New Ingredients

Any life crisis brings change on many levels. Early in the cardiac crisis the basic elements of your life-style are the most noticeably affected. At a time when you especially need nourishment and rest, you are coping with new dietary requirements and disrupted sleep. No aspect of your life is immune to this crisis. Your work schedule, leisure time, and social life have been interrupted and altered. Your primary relationship too is in transition. And your personal goals and dreams, beliefs and values, are undergoing change as a result of your mate's heart disease.

Adopting a heart-healthy diet is the number one concern for most couples in the early stage of recovery. Before you became a cardiac spouse, you were probably only vaguely aware of diets that may have prevented heart disease. You may have gradually shifted your family away from red meats and toward fish and fibers. A heart-healthy diet is not much different than the general trend toward nutritious eating. But for the cardiac spouse it involves more than wanting to be fashionable or fit. It feels like a matter of life and death. And that puts a lot of pressure on you.

Before Marsh's heart attack, our diet was primarily Midwestern: meat and potatoes. I salted liberally, and never checked frozen foods for sodium, fat, and cholesterol content. Meals, which were previously a casual affair slipped in

between our teenagers' various extracurricular activities,
became a major undertaking.
    I had to learn to cook all over again. I found myself
unhappily spending hours in the kitchen absorbed in reci-
pes, meal planning, and food preparation. It reminded me of
being a newlywed, trying to impress my husband with deli-
cious and healthy meals. I experimented with herbs and
spices to replace the deadly salt I had been warned against.
I searched for recipes that would transform broiled pike into
barbecued ribs.

There is general agreement that diet may improve
recovery and prolong a heart patient's life, but a new food
plan requires time and planning. It can't happen over night.
One extra milligram of salt in your spouse's soup will *not*
cause him to keel over on the spot! You may feel guilty
about the eating habits you have taught your family, or you
may even believe that your cooking method was a primary
cause for your spouse's heart disease. But only in recent
years has a correlation between diet and heart disease been
seriously considered. Ten years ago, "low-sodium" was
hardly a household word. So there's no reason to blame
yourself now. To cry over whole, not skim, milk, is neither
productive nor constructive.

Use your new knowledge positively now and in the
future. But don't throw away all the food in your freezer
when your mate gets home from the hospital. During a time
of crisis, when everything is upset and upsetting, you need
to take things slowly and make changes gradually. As much
as you can, let the past go, and focus on what you can do
now.

Preparing healthy meals is a way to contribute to
your mate's recovery. For many couples, making dietary
changes together can be a statement of shared commitment and an opportunity for closeness. While a cardiac diet
may seem to lack variety or spice, it offers a potential
second chance at life.

A new food plan is a positive signpost on the road to recovery, but it may unfortunately also become a dangerous detour. For some couples, changing eating habits is a source of conflict and stress. It's common for partners to disagree about strict adherence to a food plan and how significant a factor of heart disease it is, when it comes down to selecting what foods to eat.

This is one area where being a cardiac spouse is especially difficult. You want to do everything in your power to help your mate stay on a healthy diet, but your spouse is also an adult and who is responsible enough to choose what he eats wisely.

Adjusting to a rigid new diet requires effort and discipline. Most recovering heart patients take a break from the approved list of foods now and then. Certainly you will worry about your mate's commitment to a healthy diet. But everyone deserves an occasional treat.

Overly critical comments or controlling behavior may reflect your fear of losing your spouse. Arguing about food can also be a way for both of you to blow off some steam, and act out some of the stress of your situation.

Susan took a three-month leave of absence from her job as a computer programmer in order to care for her husband, Jim, who was recovering from surgery. She devoted herself to cooking delicious, healthy meals and helping Jim stick to his diet. If they were going out to eat, Susan either called ahead to check the menu or brought along a separate meal for Jim. One summer night Jim arrived home with a pint of chocolate ice cream that he proceeded to devour. Susan, bristling with anger, burst out with, "Ice cream. You may as well eat poison."

Susan's perfect recovery plan was ruined. She didn't want Jim to be deprived of pleasure, especially since it was the first time he had broken the diet since the surgery. But watching him eat ice cream made her realize how terrified she was of losing him.

Monitoring your mate's diet is your way of trying to maintain control in a situation that is overwhelming and actually beyond your control. In a time of crisis, when the usual ways of expressing love and caring are interrupted, the preparation of food takes on more significance. In most relationships, sharing food connects people emotionally. Women have been brought up to communicate their feelings and show their love by preparing and serving meals.

Many cardiac spouses say they sense a lack of appreciation for their efforts. Angelina, the cardiac spouse of a proud Italian restaurant proprietor, spent night after night making heart-healthy meals. After years of pasta in cream sauce, she assumed that Carl found the cardiac fare boring and bland. One day Angelina drove clear across town to a gourmet grocery where she bought special herbs for dinner. All through the meal she waited for Carl to comment on her "Chicken Rosemary." He ate silently. Finally, she asked. His response: "I prefer it plain."

Angelina was crushed. She interpreted Carl's reaction as a personal rejection of her and her cooking. In fact, his lack of enthusiasm probably had little to do with Angelina or her efforts to please him. More likely it was a statement about his own change in values regarding food, an indication of depression, or of his effort to cope with his new diet. (And many a recovering heart patient becomes apathetic about food, or decides that is less of a priority in life.)

During this transition, communication is every bit as important as cuisine. There is no diet plan that will assure immortality, no one way to prepare food or eat it that is right for a particular couple. But you and your mate can talk about the dietary changes that heart disease has brought to your household and negotiate how to cope with this ongoing adjustment in your lives.

FOOD ISSUES TO DISCUSS WITH YOUR HEARTMATE
Questions to ask are:

How important an issue is diet to you?
How do you feel about sticking to the diet?
Who is responsible for changing and controlling the diet?
How do you want to handle exceptions ("cheating") to the
    diet?
What can you do if the two of you disagree?
Are you willing to eat a heart-healthy diet?
How can you share responsibility for a new food plan?
How can you best take care of yourself in relation to food
    and diet?
What support do you want and need to help you with this
    diet reform?

It may be new for you to think so seriously about
how and what you eat and feed your family, but understanding your beliefs and feelings about food will prove useful.
You have the opportunity to follow a healthier food plan,
one that is more satisfying and nourishing to both of you.
Because diet is a risk factor, the emotional stress attached
to it is high. But we all have to eat, and the cardiac spouse
can choose a brand new, healthy approach to food.[1]

Getting Your Rest

In order to provide your mate with support, it is
essential for you to maintain your own health and well-
being. In caring for the patient, you may unconsciously
place your own needs for sleep and healthy eating second.
Cardiac spouses often report that they are too worried or
anxious to sleep. Interrupted or fitful sleep is a natural
reaction to stress. Once the initial numbness and shock
wear off, it is normal to remain on guard and tense. If your

whole life can change in an instant, it might happen again at any time. Your entire being responds to the continuing threat of danger. The initial crisis has passed, yet it is difficult to relax and sometimes to sleep.

There probably isn't a cardiac spouse anywhere who hasn't awakened abruptly in the middle of the night, ready to dial 911. I spent many nights holding my breath, listening for the sound of breathing, waiting anxiously to see the blanket move gently up and down. It triggered my memory of being a new mother, always listening with one ear for the baby.

Recovering cardiac patients often sleep fitfully and need naps during the day. This change may be temporary, caused by the new medications and the trauma of going through a heart attack or cardiac procedure. Irregular sleep or changes in your mate's sleeping patterns aren't necessarily danger signals or something to be concerned about. Still, it may take some time before you will be able to fall asleep peacefully, confident that your partner is all right.

You may also be worried that lack of sleep will be a setback to recovery. Having been told that rest is an essential part of the healing process may increase your anxiety about your partner's restlessness. *But worry doesn't help.* Although it took many months, I finally stopped asking my morning worry question, "How did you sleep last night?" For me, Marsh's report of how many times he had awakened in the night, or of how long he lay tossing and turning, counting and recounting the meager number of hours slept, only served to aggravate my concern. We'd both been awake, and we'd worried together, but it did nothing to improve his sleep.

Eventually, the patient's new sleep patterns will become more routine and less frightening to you. In the meantime, you need to get all of the rest you can in order to restore your emotional and physical energy. This may mean cutting back on some of your activities or taking the phone off the hook so that *you* can grab a nap. A short period of conscious relaxation (see appendix B for a visualization exercise to help you relax) or deep breathing for two to five minutes can relax tense muscles and calm nervous feelings.

A common sleep disturbance is waking each other up. It may be difficult for you to get used to sleeping in the same bed again. Some couples handle the problem by sleeping separately. Unless this is absolutely necessary, I caution against it, as it may become a permanent barrier to sleeping together. Once one of you has moved to a separate bed or another bedroom, it may be difficult to find a reason to return. The time apart may create feelings of shyness or a reluctance to ask for the physical closeness you need.

Deciding who will shop for the low-sodium items at the supermarket may be easier than expressing your need to be cuddled and held. But physical touching is very important. Just as food preparation can be a vehicle to express love, sharing the same bed is an opportunity for intimacy.

For the sake of your rest and in order to preserve your closeness, talk with your mate about the issues of sleep. Remember: you, too, have been through a crisis. It takes rest and care for *your* body and *your* heart to heal.

SLEEPING HINTS
Give yourself permission to nap during the day.
Take the phone off the hook when you rest.
Consider earplugs to protect your sleep from your mate's
    restlessness.
Don't rely on medication for sleep or relaxation.
Let go of your expectations about adequate sleep.
Don't count the minutes and hours that you sleep; let how
    you feel be your guide.
Listen to quiet music before going to bed.

Drink something warm and soothing (and decaffeinated) in
the evening.

Shifting Gears

Many of you are dealing with your spouse's sudden
or early retirement. Some heart patients are recommended
to change jobs to something less physically or psychologically demanding. Others may need to work fewer hours. Yet
85 percent of surviving heart attack victims are physically
able to return to normal activity within three to six months
after returning home.

During the early weeks of recuperation, no one
knows how complete recovery will be. I remember worrying incessantly about whether Marsh would be able to go
back to work as a full-time architect. It was excruciating to
wait, not knowing if he would be permanently disabled or
handicapped by angina. Most of all, I worried about the
uncertainty of our future. I felt especially anxious about our
financial responsibilities because we still had two adolescents at home. Like most heart attack survivors, Marsh was
fortunate to be able to return to his work after six weeks, at
first for four hours a day, and eventually full time.

I have worked with cardiac spouses who were less
fortunate. Claudia and Peter, both in their mid-fifties, were
told after bypass surgery that he should change jobs.
Selling real estate was too stressful. Before Peter's surgery,
Claudia's salary had been only supplemental. Her night job
as a nurse's aide now became their sole source of income.
As they watched their life savings dwindle, Peter and Claudia
began to feel scared and depressed. Finally they sought
professional help. In order to qualify for vocational training, Peter was classified as "disabled" by the state. He was
trained in a government rehabilitation program and, after a
full year of unemployment, finally found a job. No one
addressed what that stigma had meant to him, just as

earlier no one had considered the stress he would undergo being unemployed. Six months later, Claudia became ill and needed to have fibroid tumor surgery. Her strength through the cardiac crisis and the year of Peter's unemployment, her stability as a breadwinner and wife, had taken their toll. She became the patient and needed to be cared for.

Whether your spouse retires, changes vocation, or stays with the same job, it's important for you to be involved in making the decisions. You may hesitate to express your opinion because you don't want to add any stress. But the stress already exists. Your questions and concerns are probably very similar to your mate's.

It is *normal and stressful* for a heart patient to be concerned about what recovery really means. He asks himself any number of questions: Will pain prohibit my normal activity? Will reduced cardiac efficiency keep me from working at my regular pace? Will I have to change jobs? Will my wife respect me if I can no longer be the breadwinner? Will we be able to pay the bills with less income? What kind of sacrifices will we have to make? Discussing these issues can reduce the burden each of you is carrying alone. Together you may be able to devise a more creative plan to cope with the financial distress and the work situation. Two heads are better than one, and being supportive of each other's recovery will yield benefits to both.

Economic pressures are only one aspect of work stress during recovery. You may be involved in your own career as well as trying to facilitate your mate's recovery. It may be necessary for you to make adjustments in your work schedule or even to change jobs in order to provide for your family.

One of the hardest lessons I learned as a cardiac spouse was the importance of going on with my own life. I had to alter my work schedule to account for the changes that were happening in my personal life. At times I was too distraught to give my full attention to my therapy clients.

There were days when I felt guilty for being healthy, going off to work, and leaving Marsh at home alone. I felt uncomfortable sharing my enthusiasm and sense of accomplishment about work because I thought Marsh might feel envious or anxious about his own career. At other times, work was a refuge, a place where I didn't think about myself and I could focus on someone else. I needed to return to my work because it gave me stability and a sense of normalcy. It also helped to reduce my anxiety about our finances.

In some cases, cardiac spouses sacrifice their own careers because of their mate's heart disease. When Marjorie first came to see me, she complained of boredom. As a young, single parent, she had developed a successful management career and had raised her three children. She recalled her loneliness during those years, but her responsibilities to her children had kept her working hard, and her career success was a source of great satisfaction. She considered herself a valuable member of society.

Once her children were grown and her responsibilities lessened, she began to see Phillip, a business colleague. Although he was ten years older, they decided to marry. She had the best of both worlds: a stimulating career and a husband who was a close companion and an equal in business.

After four wonderful years together, Phillip had a seriously damaging heart attack. Marjorie decided to retire with him, although she was only fifty-three at the time. Since his cardiac crisis, Phillip and Marjorie have been inseparable. The only time they are apart is once a week, when a friend comes to take Phillip out for lunch. Marjorie misses the stimulation of her job and her old way of life. Honoring her marriage at the expense of her career, Marjorie has sacrificed an important aspect of her identity and her self-esteem. Now she is looking for something that will give her own life a broader meaning. But a life-style change is not so simple. Phillip relies heavily on her for care, attention, and security. She feels responsible for his health and worries about what will happen if there is another emergency and she is gone. She needs to find ways to give her own life meaning without jeopardizing her marriage.

Coping with work changes can be extremely stressful for both of you. There is no one right answer for any cardiac couple. It is important to discuss work issues. Avoiding them won't make them disappear. Ignoring such a sensitive topic may become the biggest problem of all. Seek professional counsel if you and your mate cannot talk about your feelings.

Discussions about work can be practical and productive. You may discover that your feelings are similar. Each of you is learning to make adjustments and redefine priorities. Once you can talk, you can brainstorm about your options. Perhaps together you can devise a plan of flexible reentry into the work force. Maybe you will find some useful projects around the house to complete during recuperation. If you talk about your mutual concerns, this recovery period can also be a time to get reacquainted as a couple, and to begin long-term planning based on your realistic appraisal of possibilities and new priorities. Sharing your concerns may somewhat ease your fears, diminish your loneliness, and allow you to work as a team.

Simple Pleasures

Obviously, your social and leisure activities have been affected by the "cardiac life-style." What before seemed like simple decisions-whether to go to a movie or play doubles tennis-become major issues in adjusting to a heart-healthy life. You want to protect your mate's health, but at the same time maintain your friendships and other interests.

When I first met Loreen, a thirty-seven-year-old cardiac spouse, she was trying to cope with changes in her social life. Six weeks after Tony's heart attack, Loreen planned a celebration barbecue for some of their friends. It was a beautiful summer evening. Everyone enjoyed the company, the good food, the new deck, and the lovely yard. Loreen felt pleased with her party and grateful that her life, so recently in chaos, was back to normal. She glanced at Tony and found him fast asleep in the lawn chair. It wasn't even dark yet! And what about their guests?

Loreen talked about how she felt that night: lonely, embarrassed, angry, and sad. She also shared her worries about her future. What other life-style limitations would she encounter? How would she control her resentment if, at thirty-seven, her social life were to be permanently restricted?

Loreen's questions are not hers alone. Many cardiac spouses wonder the same things, especially during the active recovery stage (the first three months after a heart attack or bypass surgery) as the cardiac patient regains strength through a combination of rest and graduated activity. It is not unusual for a cardiac patient to nod off occasionally, even when something interesting is happening. You may feel embarrassed or impatient if your mate drifts in and out of conversation or moves at a snail's pace. You may question his motivation or even harbor resentment that he isn't improving more quickly. You may need to alter your expectations during recovery. The cardiac patient needs time and psychological space to integrate the many changes resulting from heart disease.

There isn't anything you can do to speed up the process. However, there are ways to adapt to it. During this period, you may ask your friends to be more flexible in accommodating your needs. It is likely that they will be understanding and tolerant of the situation. A rigorous night at the bowling alley may be replaced by a quiet evening watching VCR movies and munching salt-free popcorn.

As the weeks go by and your spouse's physical recovery progresses, you may wonder when it's appropriate to return to your hobbies, avocational activities, and friendships. At what point is it okay to resume your weekly tennis game, luncheon out with friends, an evening bridge game, volunteer work, the monthly book club meet ing, or other activities you were involved in before? You may feel guilty going out and enjoying yourself when your partner is home in bed. Or you may think that the seriousness of heart disease precludes recreation and fun. Some cardiac spouses are afraid of criticism, worrying that being seen in public "having a good time" when a spouse has suffered a heart attack implies that they are insensitive, uncaring, or selfish. Others just don't feel the old enthusiasm for projects that had been important before all this began.

The decision to resume your own activities is an individual matter. It's very important to be involved in something besides caring for your recovering mate. Time for yourself, whether it's reading a book, exercising, or shopping with a friend, is an important part of this transition. Maintaining interests in other areas of your life is essential for your own needs and to restore a realistic balance to your relationship.

Every cardiac couple is different when it comes to the level of expectation for social and leisure activities. However, you can realistically expect your mate to make gradual progress and to have more energy each week.

There is the possibility that your mate sustained substantial heart damage that will permanently restrict his physical activity. You may be a marathon runner, or just a weekend jogger, but your mate may now find it difficult to walk a flight of stairs or get through dinner without being short of breath.

Some cardiac spouses give up their own physical activities to reduce the differences and avoid conflict. Others change their activities temporarily or adjust their paces to match their mates'. If you are feeling uncomfortable about exercising when it isn't an option for your partner, be sure to talk about it together. Assess your physical health and emotional well-being before making a decision based only on your spouse's condition and prognosis. Keep in mind that your choices may be short-term and that your mate's condition will continue to change.

The cardiac life-style doesn't require you to trade in your running shoes for a cane and a pair of bifocals. Set the old bedridden stereotype aside! Recent medical trends have stressed the importance of regular exercise to strengthen the cardiovascular system and the general health of the heart patient. If your spouse participates in a cardiac rehabilitation program, he will get the supervised exercise he needs as well as a support network of fellow patients.

Recovery programs usually encourage cardiac spouses to participate. Regular exercise is important for *your* physical health, too. I recommend it as an antidote for restless nights, irregular appetite, and general lack of energy. Exercise is also an activity that the two of you may enjoy doing together.

Adding regular exercise to your routine requires effort, but it will more easily become a part of your schedule if you plan physical activity together three or four times a week. Whether you walk, bike, swim, or exercise more strenuously, what's important for health is to exercise regularly. Of course, you should check any exercise plan with the doctor before you begin. And doing something special together is another opportunity for closeness and companionship.

Who Are You Now? A Question Of Identity

You can change the way you cook, and you can adjust to coming home earlier on Saturday night. You can exercise regularly, and you can learn to live with less money, and you will still be you. But the changes that cardiac spouses experience go deeper. They affect the very center of your identity.

Identity is often experienced in the roles you play in daily life. People commonly identify themselves according to their responsibilities, by what they do, not who they are. For example, I would describe my primary roles as: wife, mother, sister, friend, therapist, daughter, and writer. In addition, your identity is dictated by your beliefs about the world. If you say you are an optimist, a "people" person, or a devout Christian, you are identifying yourself in another way.

As a cardiac spouse, your roles and your beliefs are in the process of changing. From the first moment of the cardiac crisis, when you were faced with all those new responsibilities, you assumed a different behavior. While continuing to maintain your regular activities, you took charge of healthy meal planning, medication schedules, visiting hours, and keeping your family intact.

Since a cardiac crisis happens quickly and requires immediate action, it is natural to step into new roles without even noticing you're doing so. But if you stop to look, you might be surprised to see that you have taken on one or more of the following roles.

THE HEAD NURSE

Does your everyday vocabulary include words like: pulse rate, angina, edema, stress test?

Have you become an expert on the side effects of medications?

Are you constantly adding questions to your list for your next call to the doctor?

Is it difficult for you to go "off duty" and just relax with your mate?

If this sounds familiar, you may be wearing the crisp starched cap and white uniform of the Head Nurse. Although your patient load is light, it really matters. Keeping track of medications and communicating with the doctor may seem like your official duties. Even though you don't have any medical training, you feel fully responsible for your mate's recovery. Also, it may be reassuring to take on the nurse's role, because the d uties are so clearly defined. However, it can be very exhausting to feel as if your mate's health depends on your constant medical supervision. Even though there are pill bottles everywhere, your home is still your home, not a hospital. You are needed as a helpmate, not as a nurse.

THE TRAFFIC COP

Are you constantly on guard for danger?
Do you check to see if each medication is taken on time?
Do you pride yourself on your ability to make fast decisions?
Are the words "slow down" always on the tip of your tongue?

It is perfectly natural for you to want to take charge, to want to replace chaos with order. There are schedules to be followed and decisions to be made. It's important to take your responsibilities seriously. Heart disease is no laughing matter. However, it isn't necessary to acquire the stiff-brimmed hat and dress blues of the Traffic Cop. Your well-meaning efforts to keep your mate's recovery on track may have included taking an authoritative stance. It's stressful for you to be on guard all the time. And your mate may interpret your concern as control rather than support. Perhaps it's time to turn in your uniform and whistle. Guiding, not directing, traffic will be better for both of you.

THE CHEF

Have you purchased more than two new cookbooks in
    search of heart-healthy recipes?
Do you feel discouraged when your mate doesn't compli-
    ment you on your culinary skills?
Do you insist on bringing your mate's own meal from home
    when you are invited to someone's house for
    dinner?
Do you spend hours reading nutritional charts?

If creating heart-healthy meals has become your
full-time career, you may have slipped into the role of the
Chef. You constantly look for healthy delectable recipes,
hoping to aid your mate's recovery and elevate his spirits.
Being the Chef is a way for you to feel positively involved in
improving your mate's health. However, you might feel let
down if, after slaving away in the kitchen, he doesn't appear
to appreciate your efforts. If you take off your white toque
and apron, you will be less likely to set yourself up for
disappointment. Cardiac patients often aren't enthusiastic
about eating. Your mate's appetite is not a reflection of your
culinary ability or of his love.

THE MOTHER

Do you find yourself constantly worrying, wringing your
    hands, pacing back and forth?
Do you find yourself talking to your mate in a soothing and
    pacifying tone?
Is all of your attention devoted to your mate's care?
Are you afraid to leave your home in case your mate needs
    your help?

When someone you love hurts, it is natural to feel
protective. But if most of your time is spent coddling and
taking care of your mate, you may have unknowingly taken

on the role of the Mother. Mothers are known for their nonstop worrying and selfless giving. It's one reason why they're always so tired. Right now it may be necessary to do more than your usual share. But if you have a perpetually worried look on your face, you may be taking on more responsibility than is good for either of you. Treating your spouse like a youngster will only add to his feelings of helplessness. And after a while, you may begin to resent his demands. Your mate needs your help, but he doesn't need you to be his mother. And you don't need another child.

Coping with Change

As you can see by looking at all the stereotypes described above, much more than your life-style has been changed by the cardiac crisis. You may not be aware of how much your roles and identity have changed. Most people find it difficult to be objective about themselves.

This evaluation guide will help you assess the changes in your life. Many cardiac spouses have found it valuable to write their responses in a Heartmates® notebook or journal. Writing clarifies thinking; it is a safe way to express feelings and is a useful reference during later stages of recovery. Major categories of change, such as food, are listed. Following each category are guidelines to help you explore specific changes within the category. Consider each aspect as it relates to your life before and after the cardiac crisis.

HEARTMATES® ASSESSMENT OF CHANGE

Sleep	Food
Quantity	Level of appetite
Quality	Time spent shopping
Disturbances	Time spent preparing food
Dreams and nightmares	Frequency of eating out
Frequency of naps	Primary foods
	Priority in your life

Exercise

Type	Schedule and hours
Frequency	Level of satisfaction
Quantity	Quality of work
Strenuousness	
Regularity	**Financial Responsibilities**
Differences between you	Providing income
	Budgeting
Leisure Activities	Allocating funds
Types of involvement	Handling banking
Schedule and hours	
Level of satisfaction	**Friends/Social Activities**
Quality of work	Frequency
	Quality of time spent
Work/Career	Level of satisfaction
Degree of involvement	Initiating activity

Once you have an objective sense of the changes that have already occurred, you can begin to understand those with which you are satisfied or where you want to initiate further change. For example, if you notice that you have let a friendship lapse, invite someone over or plan an outing with a friend. You have the power to reach out for the support and understanding that you need. On the other hand, you may be very pleased with the modifications you've made in your diet. Your spouse's cardiac condition may have caused you to focus attention on your own physical health and your need to eat differently.

Given the unexpectedness of the cardiac crisis and the pace at which you have functioned during your partner's recovery, it may be a real relief to stop and take stock. The ability to step back and look is a good sign that you are on the road to recovery.

It may be difficult to go over financial papers, wills,

and insurance, because it acknowledges mortality. But once you have done this, you may find a sense of peace replacing the panic in your chest. Your nightmare of having to sell all your possessions will be replaced by a more realistic assessment of your earning skills. Facing your fiscal reality increases your trust in your own resilience and flexibility. If you've always left the finances to your mate, pretending you don't have a head for figures, then assuming more responsibility might increase your confidence in yourself. You might even find that you like doing the family accounting.

An essential first step in coping with change is comprehending what has happened to you, by taking an objective look at yourself and your situation. The next step is to acknowledge your strengths in dealing with the crisis thus far. It's important to recognize that you have managed to the best of your ability through a difficult time.

It isn't easy to affirm your strengths. Most of us are more comfortable with criticism than with compliments. We find it difficult to appreciate our positive qualities, and we are more aware of our weaknesses than our strengths. You may even be admonishing yourself with internal dialogue- "I should be more caring and attentive. . . I should be more worried about him . . . I shouldn't relax my vigil. . . I shouldn't feel bad, sad, or mad. . . I shouldn't have a good time or enjoy myself." And, above all, "I don't deserve to give myself any credit for handling the cardiac crisis well, because I haven't done it perfectly."

No one is perfect. But taking credit for doing your best is an important part of the recovery process. Something that has worked well for many cardiac couples is making a pact to share one thing each day that you appreciate about yourselves. In that way a realistic and ongoing assessment of your situation can continue. You will have something worthwhile to talk about with each other every day.

Continued assessment of the ongoing changes will help you recognize and accept reality. I would like to be able to tell you that the road to recovery is straight and narrow, but I know that it rarely is. The road sign reads "uncertainty," and accepting that requires a new belief in your ability to live with permanent change. For many cardiac spouses, the most difficult part of aftercare is coming to terms with uncertainty. The road is different for every cardiac spouse. For some, the road may have more potholes and unexpected turns. If you are fortunate, recovery may be a long, lasting journey, and the reality of a life with someone with heart disease may be accepted as simply as part of growing older together.

At the Heart of the Matter

I recently encountered a woman whose husband had just passed his six-month mark. I congratulated her on his recovery. She nodded thanks, but something about her expression made me wonder if she was okay. When I gently asked her, she recounted a familiar story. Ever since her husband's return from the hospital, their marriage had become increasingly stressful. Before his surgery they had been compatible and close. Now they vacillated between constant bickering and strained silence. Their home, which had always been a haven, was beginning to seem like a battleground.

This woman's story reminded me of how difficult a marriage relationship can be in the first six to twelve months of recovery. Paradoxically, there is much to be thankful for. You feel grateful beyond measure that your mate has recovered, regained strength, and is back on his feet. The image of him weak and vulnerable in the hospital is slowly fading. It's not so easy to recall fitful sleep and irregular meals, or the sense of disorientation and helplessness. You've probably acquired enough expertise about medications, diet, and the terminology that accompanies cardiac disease to run the educational program at the hospital. Your husband has not called a doctor in weeks, maybe even months.

It's a relief to settle back into a regular routine. The new order, incorporating scheduled exercise and dietary changes, is almost second nature. There is less pressure on you to care for a patient, and you have enough time for family, activities, and work. Friends and relatives have returned to their normal lives, and don't call or visit as often. Some days you don't even react when you get an unexpected telephone call or hear an ambulance siren in the night.

And yet *your* transition continues. You looked forward to celebrating your mate's recovery. Some days you feel great; other days you can't seem to pull yourself out of the doldrums. Your husband has returned to work and your family is "back to normal." *But what was normal before bears little or no resemblance to life as you know it today.*

Your life is different. There are a number of issues that make this period especially complicated. The one person you normally count on for support is emotionally out of reach. Ironically, your mate may be around more, but you feel lonelier than ever. Heart patients are, as a rule, engrossed in their physical symptoms. Even when your spouse is physically present, his preoccupation with himself may leave little room for your needs.

Your mate may also be more demanding of your time and want you to stay nearby just for security. Activities that you used to share, like volunteer work or playing in a mixed bowling league, may no longer interest him or may be out of the question because of medical limitations. If your routine keeps you at home with your recovering spouse, the increased proximity may limit your mobility and freedom. You may even begin to feel smothered, as if you are losing yourself in this entity called heart disease.

Your relationship with your spouse has changed in both obvious and subtle ways. No one has a perfect marriage. But you probably consider your spouse one of the half dozen people you are closest to in the world. Before the cardiac crisis you may have told him about things that were important to you. You probably discussed opinions and issues on a regular basis. You may have shared inner secrets, hopes, and dreams. At times, you experienced regular physical closeness and sexual intimacy. You felt a connection partially made up of years spent together-living, working, and raising a family.

The onset of the cardiac crisis caused a major break in your relationship. First there was the physical separation; you slept at home while he, surrounded by medical equipment and strangers, slept in the hospital. Then there was a breakdown in communications. The shock of the crisis made you unsure of what to say or how to respond. You got the message that your spouse needed rest and shouldn't experience stress. You wore makeup to cover the dark circles under your eyes, a product of stress and sleeplessness, and you were the cheerleader who encouraged him on the short, slow walk down the hospital corridor. You tried to act cheerful and upbeat when you really felt worried and sad. You held back your tears so that he wouldn't be burdened by your anguish. The more you disguised your feelings, the greater the distance grew between you.

For some couples, there is a carry-over of that emotional distance into the recovery phase and beyond. You may still be as withdrawn as you were when you stood at his hospital bedside. Your communication with each other may be stilted for fear of creating stress or making each other feel worse. You may even believe that your relationship is so fragile that it will begin to fall apart if you start talking.

You may not be aware of the energy it takes to hide your feelings from your mate. And, in the long run, you are setting up a mode of communication that inhibits rather than promotes honesty in your marriage. Your mate may wonder what really lies beneath your cheerful countenance or resent your apparent confidence when he is feeling so scared. Besides, he needs to be needed now, too. Why not break down the barriers by reaching out to each other? There is an old adage that goes: "When you share joy it is doubled; when you share pain it is halved. "

Those Powerful Feelings

Feelings are your reaction to the world around you. Your feelings are the normal and predictable responses to the cardiac crisis you have experienced. You need to acknowledge and respect them as real and important.

It's natural to put off dealing with your feelings in the height of the emergency. But the emergency is over! And your feelings have not disappeared. In fact, some of them are stronger. It is harder to ignore and control them as the weeks and months pass. They get in the way and intensify what is already a difficult situation between you and your mate. Trying to control your feelings takes a great deal of energy, and may strain your relationship with your mate beyond the original crisis.

Though he may not have expressed it, your spouse is struggling with similar feelings. Most of the professional attention he received concentrated on his physical care. Friends focus their encouragement on tangible aspects of recovery like improved endurance and increased strength. But the depth of the emotional, mental, and spiritual crisis the cardiac patient weathers is often unrecognized.

Remember your spouse has to make emotional adjustments while he copes with the physical realities of heart disease. Most likely, it is a struggle for him to accept what has happened. Facing physical limitations, heart patients are prone to volatile feelings. Some patients manifest their anger by being demanding, withdrawn, irritable, or overly solicitous. Others demonstrate their fear by denying that anything has changed. They may act out by continuing to smoke and eat the wrong foods. They may lift heavy objects, return to work without permission from their physician, or push physical limits until they're exhausted. One woman insisted on vacuuming and scrubbing her kitchen floor one month after bypass surgery. She admitted to being independent and stubborn. But she was also unwilling to limit herself or care wisely for herself, even before her incision pain had disappeared.

Most of us find it difficult to step into another person's emotional shoes. When you are in the midst of an intense experience, you cannot readily identify and empathize with anyone else's feelings. But you ought to try to understand what your mate is going through for two reasons: so you can see how his attitude and behavior are affecting you, and so you can begin to support each other. Your spouse's physical heart has healed, and you need not fear damaging it by stating your feelings and concerns.

Feelings can be divided into two general categories: positive and negative, experienced as pleasurable and painful. When you experience a crisis, you suffer an emotional wound. It's common for people to try to avoid or ignore the resulting painful feelings. When something happens that is beyond personal control, people move unconsciously to what is familiar. The most common reaction is to fall back on habitual behavior.

Most of us like to think of ourselves as kind, open, and loving. We find it more difficult to accept our anger and disappointment. Guilt, fear, and sadness may be more familiar, but they can be overwhelming. All of these feelings are appropriate responses to the intense changes you have experienced. If you're like most cardiac spouses, you may have thought, or even voiced, something like: "I'm trying to do everything right, but I can't stop crying. . . I'm snapping at everyone all the time. . . It's so hard to keep my hopes up when I'm so worried. . . I'm afraid I'm coming apart, and I don't know what to do about it."

All of these feelings are normal. Give yourself permission to have all of your feelings, including the "negative" ones, and you will be more able to do something about them. The first step is to recognize what they are.

Anxiety, the Great Paralyzer

Cardiac spouses experience profound fears. What are they, and why are they so powerful? You have been thrown abruptly into a situation that threatens all aspects of your life. Once the initial terror passes, you are faced with the great unknown. Before the cardiac crisis you felt relatively secure and sure of yourself. Now you feel anxious and uncertain about the future.

Anxiety is defined as the fear of being hurt or losing something. All cardiac spouses are afraid of losing their partners. This kind of fear manifests itself in thinking of foreboding questions without any answers. During the interminable hours you waited outside the hospital emergency room, wondering whether your mate was still alive, close to death, resting comfortably, or in excruciating pain, you undoubtedly asked yourself: What are the chances for survival? Perhaps your anxiety was most acute at the beginning of the crisis, when everything was "touch and go." Or perhaps your numbness might have protected you, whereas now you are haunted by questions of survival. In either case, the terrible fear of being widowed doesn't evaporate the minute your mate is discharged from the hospital. Surgical success and cardiac rehabilitation aside, no heart patient is given a clean bill of health. Consequently, all cardiac spouses live with the anticipation and fear of a fatal episode. Your anxiety can be provoked quickly and easily. Think about how you feel when your spouse cuts your regular walk short without telling you why. Consider your reaction when you see him "popping nitros," checking his pulse, or taking his blood pressure.

Emily was called long distance and informed that her husband had suffered a heart attack. He was in a strange city, halfway across the country, where he was attending a sales show. Emily and Theo had no family in their city to take care of their two young daughters, but Emily quickly made emergency arrangements with a friend, and flew off to support and help care for Theo.

Terrified and alone in a motel in a strange city, Emily had to rely on the advice of strangers. She slept poorly, ate hurriedly in coffee shops, and spent as much time as she could with Theo in a strange hospital.

It was frightening, lonely, and stressful to spend each day in the hospital and to return to a motel room each night. Having to function as an optimistic messenger for Theo's worried parents and their own frightened children, Emily quickly exhausted much of her energy. As Theo's recovery progressed, a nurse gave Emily explicit instructions about getting him home safely, and caring for him once there. She advised purchasing first-class seats on the airplane, and arranging for wheelchair support at the airport to meet Theo at the gate when they arrived.

Finally they were on their way home. Just before landing, the flight attendant came over to them, leaned toward Theo, and said, "The wheelchair for your wife is at the gate, so don't worry." Emily's fear had taken so great a toll that she was mistaken for the cardiac patient who needed special care.

The fear of losing your mate escalates if he doesn't seem committed to recovery. His seemingly cavalier attitude may frustrate you. You simply don't trust his good judgment about how much he can do. Anxiety mounts as you see that your mate hasn't stopped smoking or that he is gaining weight. How can you help but panic when he insists on shoveling snow, moving furniture, lifting heavy boxes, or jogging too far? It isn't unusual for heart patients to test their limits: to prove something to themselves or to feel useful and needed. Men may feel added pressure to reassert their masculinity. Whatever the reason, it adds up to more anxiety for you.

Most people experience anxiety as a combination of physical symptoms mixed with an overwhelming sense of helplessness. In cases of severe anxiety, you may feel uneasy, unsettled, or even agitated. Your heartbeat may speed up and "butterflies" may flutter in your stomach. You may shake or tremble uncontrollably, sweat, get cold feet and hands. Less intense reactions include tense muscles, tightening of neck and shoulders, clenched teeth, and a vague sense of impending loss.

I remember the terror. It began about the time Marsh was due to leave the hospital. I was terrified that he would die at any moment now that we were away from the doctor and the nursing staff; terrified that he'd never recover enough to resume his place in the family as husband, father, and breadwinner; terrified that I wouldn't have the inner strength to care for him, to maintain my responsibilities as the new leader of the family. I was terrified that I felt so alone and no one seemed to know, and terrified that now that Marsh was home everyone would abandon us, believing we no longer needed their support or help. And, most of all, I was terrified that just thinking this way proved that I was crazy, abnormal, or that I had cracked under the pressure.

Another fear expressed by many cardiac spouses is that of being abandoned, being left alone. For a younger cardiac spouse it may evoke fears of inadequacy, of inability to raise children alone. But, for older cardiac spouses, whose children have grown and left home, the thought of being widowed can be even worse. Merriam, a seventy-year-old cardiac spouse, remarried late in life. After losing her first husband to heart disease, Merriam raised their two children alone. Once they were grown, she began to see an old high school sweetheart, a widower. They married in their middle sixties, largely out of need for security and companionship. Merriam's second husband recently suffered a heart attack, and now Merriam has become terrified of abandonment. She finds it difficult to express her anxiety about aging and dying alone.

Since men experience heart disease earlier in life than most women, the majority of cardiac spouses are female. Older women are particularly vulnerable to financial survival fears, because a large percentage have worked exclusively as homemakers. Financial decisions are especially difficult during a time of crisis. Becoming a "bag lady" is a very real specter for many women. Others describe nightmares about the mortgage company appearing on the doorstep with the threat of foreclosure.

Although I have worked for most of my adult years, I felt terrified about finances after Marsh's heart attack. My thinking, repetitious and negative, went something like this: "There's no way we can keep the house, we'll have to sell it. The kids have been so happy here. They'll hate living in a small apartment. There's probably not an apartment in this neighborhood that we can afford. The kids will have to change schools. How will I ever put them through college on my income alone?"

One morning, my terror got the best of me. I called the social security office to ask how much money each of our children would get if Marsh died or was permanently disabled. Never mind that his heart attack had been described as minor by the doctor or that his recovery so far had been uncomplicated.

I was distraught. I needed information to calm me down, but then I struggled with another fear: Had I put a hex on Marsh's recovery? By thinking about money, disability,

*and death, I might have caused the very outcome I dreaded
most, in a sort of self-fulfilling prophecy!*

Chronic anxiety is common in situations where
heart disease is severe and increasingly debilitating. When
Edith first came to me, she needed help managing her
overwhelming fears. Her husband, Richard, had suffered
several heart attacks, bypass surgery, and almost every
possible complication. Edith explained that she had called
911 numerous times over the last six years. She actively
worried every time she left the house, dreading another
emergency, convinced that she wouldn't be there to save
him. Her stomach and head ached, her muscles were tight,
her speech was clipped, and her movements were agitated
and jumpy. She felt frantic each time she watched Richard
take his pulse or heard him sigh audibly.

Edith was disappointed in herself because she
couldn't control—or get rid of—her fear. She equated
courage with fearlessness. When we talked about how
strong she had been during the six years she cared for
Richard, she said that fear had never stopped her from
acting quickly or resolutely. And once Edith was able to
appreciate her courage, she began to accept her fears.

When she hears Richard cough or sigh, Edith still
experiences fear. But now, before her fears race ahead in
her thoughts to a catastrophic conclusion, she takes a deep
breath and says to herself: "I feel afraid and I have my
courage." This helps her keep her fear from escalating, and
reminds her of her strength.

The first step in dealing with anxiety is the hardest:
You must admit that you are afraid. Fear is like an alarm that
alerts us to defend and protect ourselves in a threatening
situation. If you ignore your anxiety and pretend that
everything is fine, you will spend energy you really can't
afford and in no way alleviate your fear.

Once you recognize that you feel anxious, you need
to ask yourself, "What am I afraid of losing?" Try to be very

specific. Deal directly with the threat—do not ignore or deny it—and perceive your situation anew. You can then choose to accept what you cannot change, and plan ways to act on what you can change.

As you face your fears, it is equally important to take stock of your strengths, those qualities you can count on in yourself during an emergency or a difficult time. Look specifically at the cardiac crisis you have been through, and be sure to recognize what you have done well. View your strengths as an advantage in your plan to change what can be changed; they'll help you succeed.

Why not ask a friend or relative to listen to your fears? Let your confidante know that you don't expect her to fix things, that what you need is an ear, and maybe a shoulder. Sometimes anxiety can be so severe or so prolonged that professional help, including anti-anxiety medication, is needed. Don't hesitate to consult your own physician if you find yourself unable to handle your anxiety.

Repeat the Serenity Prayer to yourself whenever you feel the need. It can be a powerful antidote to fear:

God,
grant me the serenity to
accept the things I cannot change,
the courage to change the things
I can,
and the wisdom to know the difference.

The Ogre, Anger

Are you irritated, impatient, or resentful more frequently now than before the cardiac crisis? Do you find yourself yelling at no one in particular? Are you aggravated easily for no obvious reason? If so, you are experiencing feelings of anger as do most cardiac spouses.

There are a variety of underlying reasons for your feelings of anger. Family and friends are likely to focus on the ailing cardiac patient, forgetting that you, too, are in a time of crisis. You may feel angry at the abundance of attention that your husband receives. You certainly don't begrudge him that much-needed support, but it would be nice if occasionally someone recognized *your* needs.

You may feel angry at the professional team that cared for your spouse at the hospital, or be dissatisfied with the quality of services. One woman, a cardiac nurse by profession, was furious that certain drugs weren't administered to her husband. A receptionist who has put you on hold, a doctor in a hurry, or a distracted nurse who forgets to say hello are likely targets, even scapegoats, for your anger.

It is not unusual to feel angry or irrationally agitated about something as vague or abstract as heredity or genes. This is especially true if your spouse is a non-smoker who has been exercising and eating well for years. Some cardiac spouses resent their mates for having heart attacks and disrupting their lives. Others feel irritated at their spouse for not appearing to appreciate their efforts. Still others are angry at their partners for being insensitive to their feelings during this difficult time.

Josie, a cardiac spouse, described a family holiday scene. She, her husband, and their three young sons spent Thanksgiving with relatives. Even though Jack was scheduled to undergo bypass surgery the following Monday, Josie was determined to make the holiday as pleasant as possible. All afternoon members of the family crowded around Jack, asking how he was doing and giving him their best wishes. He was the star attraction, and most of the conversation centered around his illness and impending surgery. As the day wore on Josie became first irritated and then furious. She had desperately wanted Thanksgiving to be normal, especially for the sake of their children. She felt as if her life would never again be free from the focus on heart disease.

Cardiac spouses also feel angry because their own needs for support are sorely neglected. Everyone expresses concern for the patient. Rarely does anyone remember to ask about you. One man reported feeling like a newscaster responsible for giving up-to-the-minute reports on his wife's condition. One evening, after several such phone reports, he remembered thinking that if one more person called and asked, "How's Kathryn doing?" he would slam the phone down. He just needed someone to say, "How are *you* doing, Ken? I bet this is a really difficult time for *you*." Ken felt so angry that he was tempted to disconnect the phone. What he really needed was some warm, human connection for himself.

If you are accustomed to relying on your spouse to meet many of your emotional needs, your feelings of neglect may well be exacerbated. You're not getting the affection or support you need right now. You deeply miss your partner's interest in you, your daily activities, and your thoughts and ideas. Even if he were outgoing and openly affectionate before, he may now be self-centered and engrossed with his health. It seems that every time you look, he's checking his pulse, weighing himself, or taking his blood pressure. Despite your best efforts to sympathize and understand, you still feel angry at his apparent loss of interest in you and, possibly, his lack of appreciation.

So, where do you direct your feelings? Many cardiac spouses find it impossible to feel anger toward the patient. They unconsciously deny their anger out of loyalty, confusion, fear, or guilt. When this happens, that same anger may be transferred to the doctor, nursing staff, Fate, or even God. Or you may turn the anger inward, and berate yourself for not trying to make your husband quit smoking or stop working so hard.

Attempting to explain or justify your anger is fruitless. Feelings just aren't rational. Rationalizing them is like asking yourself if it is all right to be hungry or thirsty. Like hunger and thirst, feelings exist and are normal responses to your situation. You don't need to justify your feelings to yourself or to anyone else. Your anger is a signal that you are experiencing a crisis. Use that angry energy to see that your needs are met.[1]

Getting angry is *not* dangerous to your spouse's health. Of course, I'm not suggesting that you berate your mate during the first forty-eight hours after a heart attack. Nor do I advocate that you take advantage of the situation to act like a nasty ogre, spoiled brat, or a whining witch. Both you and your mate are experiencing angry feelings about all the changes that heart disease has created in your lives. Anger doesn't mean you don't love each other. You can find appropriate ways to express your anger and learn how to diffuse it, freeing yourself to move on.

There are many ways to express anger safely and appropriately. Some people release their anger physically. You can pound the wall, swim laps vigorously, or smash a tennis- or racquetball. Some people rid themselves of anger by writing. Yell into a pillow or shout in the shower—just raising your voice is a great release.

Direct communication is the most effective way to express anger to your mate. If this is threatening or unprecedented, begin by negotiating rules for the discussion. Rules provide safety and a foundation on which to build further communication.

- Set a time limit (five minutes may be sufficient) for each of you to speak.
- Name a place that is completely private.
- Make a pact that allows honest expression of anger.
- Take turns.
- Agree not to interrupt.
- Commit to listening fully and openly.
- Remember that you are on the same team and that you love each other.

Here is a list of "do's" and "don'ts" to help you express your anger.

HEARTMATES® ANGER CHECKLIST

DO	DON'T
Do say what hurts	Don't avoid talking about important issues
Do begin all angry statements with "I"	Don't use your anger to blame
Do use your anger to clear the air	Don't use your anger to attack or punish your mate
Do try to make yourself understood	Don't mistake anger for violence or aggression
Do tell it straight	Don't exaggerate, whine, or complain
Do say what you think	Don't rationalize or intellectualize
Do say regularly how you feel	Don't save up little irritations until your anger explodes
Do raise your voice until you're heard	Don't withdraw because you'll injure your mate
Do take responsibility; "own" your anger	Don't believe your relationship is too fragile to bear the weight of your feelings
Do say you're angry	Don't sacrifice your anger in exchange for physical symptoms like headaches, depression, or ulcers

Sadness, the Heavy Weight

It may seem strange to feel sad at a time like this. Your mate is recovering. Shouldn't you be happy? Yes, but major life changes are also accompanied by feelings of sadness, even depression.

We all tend to take our lives for granted. When something happens that jeopardizes our security, we experience enormous feelings of loss. In a cardiac crisis, all that you hold near and dear has been threatened. The everyday freedom and long-term security you count on suddenly seems tenuous, or even lost.

You may recognize sadness by its effects on your body. The physical counterparts of sadness sometimes appear as lethargy or fatigue. Cardiac spouses often attempt to hide their sadness for fear of appearing ungrateful, selfish, or spoiled. In the hospital and during the recovery period, you may have "put on a happy face," and worn a mask of cheerfulness and confidence.

As you relax your pose, you may become depressed. Symptoms of depression can creep up slowly, or hit you early and hard. Depression saps your energy and reduces your ability to function. For some time , you may feel as if nothing matters or that it takes all of your stamina just to get through the day. You may even begin to question the meaning and purpose of your life.

Janet, age thirty-nine, described her life before her husband's heart attack. She jokingly referred to herself as the "Tour Director." She was constantly organizing social activities for the two of them and their friends. They were enthusiastic sports fans and patrons of the repertory theater and local art museum. They made several business trips and took vacations each year. Making arrangements was almost a full-time job for Janet. Since Brendan's bypass surgery, Janet wanders through her immaculate condominium pondering the purpose of her life. The structure of her daily routine has toppled. Accustomed to organizing and taking charge, Janet feels lost, aimless, and adrift. She is wary of feeling sorry for herself because she has always felt so privileged. But her old life is gone. Her new life is still a question mark. The void leaves her feeling empty and confused.

Few cardiac spouses have lost such an exciting and romantic way of life, but all confront the disappointment of broken dreams. Margaret, a careful and conservative person and her husband, Patrick, planned to realize a lifelong dream and retire to a quiet, rural town somewhere in a warm climate. Just one year before retirement from his construction job, Patrick suffered a severe heart attack. Their savings have dwindled because of medical and related expenses. Margaret empathizes with Patrick's fear and understands his need to stay in Wisconsin where his doctor and family members can give him the support he needs. Still, she mourns her retirement cottage in the sun.

If your mate has a second heart attack or a setback in recovery requiring angioplasty or bypass surgery, both of you may feel more disappointed than you did at the onset of the cardiac crisis. Physical recovery may be more prolonged and your depression more difficult to overcome. It takes more effort to feel optimistic and to trust in the medications, in your recovery program, even in your doctor.

Some of the sadness that cardiac spouses report indicates yearning for things past: Christmas like it used to be when he dressed up like Santa to pass out gifts to the grandchildren; those few years comparatively free of responsibility after the children were grown and before her heart attack; long driving trips through the Northwest every summer until his bypass surgery. Each holiday, every season marked from the onset of heart disease, is an occasion for gratitude *and* mourning.

I remember the audible sigh of relief when a cardiologist, speaking to a group of patients and spouses, acknowledged that it is *normal* for cardiac patients to experience depression. *The same is true for cardiac spouses.* In order to deal with depression, you must first acknowledge your sadness and disappointment. Facing your sadness may seem difficult and painful, even fearful. But disregarding it won't make it disappear. In fact, just the opposite is true. Once you accept that your feelings are legitimate, the terror will lessen. By allowing yourself to experience your sadness, you will gain faith in your resilience and confidence in your courage.

You need to let yourself grieve over your losses. This means mourning what *is* lost and can't be retrieved. It also means you must accept what is beyond your personal control. Mourning is a process, and you need to give yourself plenty of time to grieve. Don't feel that you have to be finished with your sadness or disappointment on anyone else's schedule. Don't be pressured by comments about "dwelling on your sadness" or implications that you should "hurry up and get on with your life."

One Sunday afternoon about two months after Marsh's heart attack, a friend called to invite me to the movies. It sounded like a perfect thing to do to get away. When it was time to get ready, I felt exhausted and wondered why I had agreed to the outing. I was surprised and disturbed to find that I could not keep my mind on the movie. Everyone in the theater laughed out loud, but I didn't find the clever repartée funny at all. I couldn't concentrate on or analyze the ideas presented in the film. Perhaps it was just too early for me to enjoy myself. But in the grand scheme of things, the movie seemed trivial in comparison with my personal struggles.

Our society supports quick decisions and avoidance of pain.[2] Remember that each individual is unique and experiences grief differently and at an individual pace.

When Henry David Thoreau suggested that each person hears a different drummer and needs "to step to the music which he hears, however measured or far away,"[3] he might well have been honoring the recovery of the cardiac spouse.

You may be tempted to minimize or deny your own sadness on the pretense of sacrifice or good will, but it's a myth that "acting happy" will help your mate move through his depression more quickly. And it is absolutely not true that feeling bad is a sign of weakness, craziness, or failure. Expressing your sadness doesn't negate your feelings of gratitude that your mate is recovering. And, as the New Testament (Matthew 5:4) tells us, "Blessed are those who mourn, for they shall be comforted."

In time, your sadness will diminish. You'll know naturally when you've mourned enough. Your physical, emotional, and mental energy will return. You may suddenly feel motivated to do things that for months have seemed impossible. You will find yourself spontaneously interested in others again. Your focus will shift from yearning for a lost past to planning for your future.

The Grasp of Guilt

Guilt is a complicated feeling. Sometimes it is explained as anger turned in on yourself. It's no wonder so many cardiac spouses feel guilty. What kind of a woman would feel angry at a husband who's sick and almost died? But, again, feelings aren't rational, and your anger is real. With no one else to blame, you became angry at yourself.

Guilt is sometimes used to cover up other less "acceptable" feelings. You may feel guilty because you think your feelings are selfish, wrong, or different than what is expected. All around you are well-wishers cheering for your mate's recovery. What kind of a person would risk sabotaging the patient's progress by expressing worry or fear? What sort of individual feels sad and depressed when everyone else is being cheerful and optimistic?

Guilt comes when you realize you've done something hurtful to another person and feel disappointed in yourself. Many cardiac spouses feel responsible for their mate's heart disease or heart attacks. Louise, an assertive and outspoken woman, suffered guilt for many months because she and John had been arguing when his chest pain began. As she waited and watched in the hospital, she became convinced that if she hadn't raised her voice, hadn't felt so righteous about expressing her opinion, her darling John would not be in cardiac care. Even the lectures she attended at the hospital which helped define risk factors and methods of prevention did nothing to free Louise from her belief that she had caused John's heart attack. She couldn't look at the scar on John's chest, because it was such a powerful reminder of her fault.

Louise's case may seem extreme, but consider all the ways you feel responsible. You may feel guilty for using so much salt in your cooking over the last forty years. One man felt guilty because he agreed to drive his wife to the hospital rather than call 911. He believed that the damage to his wife's heart was increased because he lost precious minutes en route. Many spouses feel guilty because they didn't try to intervene in their mate's hospital care. Still others suffer because they initiate intervention and are unsuccessful. This was dramatized in the television movie "Heartsounds" (adapted from Martha Weinman Lear's book of the same title) when a cardiac spouse confronted the night nurse to persuade her to awaken the intern to change orders. The nurse refused because she was afraid she'd lose her job.

Although you probably know that you "did the best you could in those circumstances," or realize that blaming yourself is unreasonable, it doesn't make guilt automatically disappear. Guilt becomes a problem when we don't understand it. If you feel guilty about your feelings, focus on them. Find out where your anger is coming from. Understand how *you* have been hurt. Examine your sadness and disappointment and experience those feelings fully.

If you feel guilty about hurting your spouse, assess your realistic responsibility.[4] Be accountable for your actions; apologize and make appropriate amends if the situation permits. Remember: your spouse's physical heart has healed. Your thoughts and feelings will not damage it.

A FEW POINTS TO REMEMBER ABOUT FEELINGS

• Feelings exist. You are not responsible for how you feel.
• It is *normal* to experience anger, fear, sadness, and guilt in response to the cardiac crisis.
• Recognizing and identifying your feelings relieves and empowers you.
• Feelings provide an important source of information about yourself and your reactions to the world around you.
• Feelings change over time.
• Accepting and understanding your feelings gives you options about how and when to express them.
• Your feelings make you human, unique, and individual.
• Feelings connect you to other human beings.

Working with Changing Feelings

In a crisis, it is easy to be overwhelmed by your emotions. It may be difficult to sort out your feelings, much less do anything about them. This exercise will help you understand and cope with your feelings:

Step 1: First, you must recognize *what* you are feeling. By labeling your feelings, one by one, you can begin to clarify them.

Step 2: The next step is figuring out what you need. What would help to reduce your feelings of anger, fear, and sadness?

Step 3: The third and most crucial step involves coming up with solutions. How can you help yourself? Once you know what you need, *you can take action.* Creative solutions require imagination and a positive attitude.

One way to keep yourself on track with this exercise is to put it all down in writing. I suggest you use a Heartmates® Feelings and Needs Assessment Diary daily or at least regularly for a period of weeks. As your feelings and needs change over a period of time, you may find a weekly, and then monthly, evaluation sufficient. The pages of your diary may follow the form I suggest here:

HEARTMATES® FEELINGS AND NEEDS ASSESSMENT DIARY[5]

Feelings	Needs	Solutions

Under Feelings, write down a feeling you are having that is bothering you. (Begin the sentence with "I feel...")

Under Needs, write down a need you have that is related to that feeling. (Begin the sentence with "I need... ")

Under Solutions, write down as many actions as you can think of that can satisfy your need. (Begin each sentence with "I could...")

Here are some sample entries:

• I *feel* scared about money . . . I *need* information about our health benefits . . . I *could* call our accountant; I *could* call the social security office; I *could* look at our budget and financial records from last year; I *could* ask my husband to discuss our financial situation with me.

• I *feel* irritable about everything . . . I *need* some time for myself . . . I *could* take a nap; I *could* stay out of the kitchen and go to a restaurant for dinner tonight; I *could* weed my garden; I *could* sit down and read my favorite magazine; I *could* take a warm bubble bath; I *could* go for a long walk in the park.

• I *feel* afraid of being alone . . . I *need* to belong . . . I *could* call one of our kids to arrange a visit ; I *could* take a walk with my spouse; I *could* go to lunch with my best friend; I *could* reach out to talk to my next door neighbor; I *could* arrange to do some volunteer work with others through my church or community center.

• I *feel* sad . . . I *need* to allow and express my feelings . . . I *could* have a good cry; I *could* write a sad poem; I *could* ask my mate to hold me in his arms; I *could* share my sadness with a dear friend.

The Heartmates® Feelings and Needs Assessment Diary doesn't include space for the last step in the process. This is to *choose* one of your solutions and do it. Do whatever is necessary to make your solution a reality; it's always the final step in the process.

Very often the last step involves asking for what you want from other people. For most of us, this is the hardest part. But if you are willing to reach out—to your mate, to other family members, to friends—you will have a better chance of having your need for human support met.

Seeking Support

Working your way through a crisis is a highly personal experience. How many times have you sat up late at night worrying about your mate's health and wondering about your future? You may have thought that no one understands what you're going through. You're right. It's impossible for anyone to completely comprehend your experience. But that doesn't mean that no one cares.

There are times when solitude is exactly what you need. The soul-searching done when you are alone can be peaceful and healing. But you also need support. When you are hurting, it is especially important to allow yourself to be cared for. Each of us finds comfort in different ways. Express your fear and frustration to someone who is willing to listen patiently without making judgments. The kind word or warm hug you receive in return can be a much-needed gift of support. Or you may take solace from simply being in the company of a close friend.

Your friends and family may or may not be as supportive as you'd like. Even those who try their best may fail to offer their support in the right way. Despite their good intentions, they may unwittingly contribute to your sense of isolation. Early in the crisis, friends and family are apt to check in often. Their first question is about your partner's health. And rightly so. They express relief that he's doing well and recovering quickly. Most conversations end with the statement, "You must be thrilled that everything is going so well." Their concern is appreciated, but it's hardly an invitation to express your needs.

It's not so easy to ask a friend or relative for support, especially when they don't offer it directly. If your relationship is not characterized by sharing and intimacy, you may feel uncomfortable exposing your vulnerability and asking for help. But try your best to realize that this is an extraordinary situation. The normal rules of etiquette don't apply. Your friends and family may be unsure of the appropriate way to approach you. Perhaps they too present a cheerful face in order to keep up your spirits—and their own.

If you feel uneasy expressing your feelings, experiment a little, test the waters. Share one personal thing the next time a friend, relative, or neighbor calls. Once the initial barrier is broken, it will be easier to do so again. Or make it a habit to share something once each day. Assess how it goes. Don't overdo it; take small steps.

Accepting offers of meals or even financial aid from relatives is another way of letting them be there for you. Asking a friend to stop over for an hour so that you can take a break is not an imposition in a time of crisis. If you take the risk, and ask for support, you may be pleasantly surprised by how eagerly it's given. And someday you may have the opportunity to return the favor.

Reaching Out

The best kind of support is reaching out to someone who is going through a similar experience. Other cardiac spouses are uniquely capable of relating to your feelings.

On the day of Marsh's surgery, I shared the waiting room with another cardiac spouse and her family. As the minutes crawled by, we each sat silently, alone with our thoughts. Finally, the door opened. The chaplain walked over and stood in front of me . Placing his hand on my shoulder, he said, "Your husband has come through fine; the surgery is over." My eyes filled with tears of relief. And through my tears, I saw that the other cardiac spouse was weeping, too.

During that seemingly unending block of time, we shared an intimacy that I'll never forget. The experience of the strong bond which developed so quickly between us forcefully reminded me that I was not alone. Later we kept each other company outside Intensive Care and visited each other's husband in the post surgical unit. Once we left the hospital we went our separate ways. But, in a very special way, we will always be connected.

One way to meet other cardiac spouses is to attend educational programs sponsored by your local hospital or clinic. In addition, your community may offer mental health programs that specialize in treating people affected by disease or trauma. Professional counseling during a time of crisis can be an important means of support. Contact with professionals who are sensitive to your needs may help you to cope with your loneliness and confusion.

Ultimately, *you are not alone.* Reaching out for support is an absolutely essential step in recovery and in the process of reclaiming your health — and your life.

Keeping Your Head on Straight

*T*he cardiac crisis plays havoc with your mind. From the very first instant, everything feels as though it's happening in double time. In a state of shock, you try desperately to clear your head and make the right moves. Inundated with information and advice, you struggle to make sense of it all.

A crisis affects the workings of your mind every bit as much as your feelings. As you try to comprehend what's happened, you may be surprised by your inability to think straight. It is common for cardiac spouses to have trouble concentrating and staying focused. Your ability to retain and comprehend information is affected, and you may feel as if your thoughts are crazy or out of control.

In the first days after Marsh's heart attack, my mind seemed to have a life of its own. Over and over I was plagued by a litany of unanswerable questions. Instead of thinking, "Well, I can see I'm in an awful situation, I need to figure out what to do," I was fixated on the same material, my mind like a race car careening wildly around a speedway.

The logical questions I wish I could have asked were: "What is the priority here? What do I need to think about?

What do I need to ask? What do I need to plan? What do I need to do?"

In any crisis it's hard to think, but you face an additional pressure: the difficult task of making immediate life-or-death decisions alone. Cardiac spouses, who are used to sharing decision making, now must do so without the input and support of their mates. There are pressing medical decisions to be made. At the onset of the crisis, when your mind is least functional, you are forced to act quickly and decisively.

Just hours after her husband's bypass surgery, as she was about to leave for home to get some much-needed rest, Helen was approached by her husband's medical team. They requested her permission to take Dennis back into surgery because of some unexpected internal bleeding. Overwhelmed by a sense of responsibility for his life, Helen could barely think, much less make one more decision. Through her blur of exhaustion, she summoned what was left of her energy and signed the papers.

We are generally advised to avoid decision making during a crisis. *Cardiac spouses should put off decisions except for urgent problems that require immediate attention.* Premature decisions can be costly. Any change or decision that can be avoided in a crisis situation will reduce the stress and shock that the cardiac spouse, patient, and family are already suffering.

After Carol's fifty-four-year-old husband, Bill, suffered a cardiac arrest, he was advised that he would need to spend the rest of his life in a nursing home. Carol was horrified at the idea but too distraught to protest. Like a zombie, she filled out the admittance forms. Bill was transferred from the hospital to the nursing home. Ten days later, he was literally climbing over the sides of his bed to use the bathroom. By this time, Carol had her wits about her. She and Bill decided that he should move back home and arrange for the assistance of a home health nurse, attend intensive physical therapy sessions, and participate in a cardiac rehabilitation program.

Directing Communications

No matter how you try to prevent it, you will out of necessity become the clearinghouse for news of your husband's condition. It is a task which requires a clear head. Everyone—his parents, your children, your parents, friends, his boss and coworkers—must be informed. You need to analyze very carefully what to tell whom and when. There just isn't any way to soften bad news. Some cases are pretty straightforward; others are more sensitive.

My most delicate call was to Marsh's mother. Who would be more worried than his mother? Widowed twenty years ago when her husband died after a heart attack, she too has heart disease. I was afraid that the shock might aggravate her condition.

I had to be careful about when to call (certainly not at midnight when he was diagnosed). Luckily, Marsh's condition was not so critical that I couldn't wait for morning. Then, there was the question of how much to say. At that point I hadn't been given any test results or a prognosis. I wanted to give her an accurate picture without alarming her unnecessarily.

Comprehending the seriousness of the situation is another extremely difficult and draining task. Family members in other parts of the country may ask *you* to decide whether *they* should "be there." The complexities of family relationships make this a touchy issue. Your spouse may want to see some relatives, but not others. You are the designated spokesperson in the unenviable, uncomfortable position of having to say yes or no. You must be tactful, yet continue to respect your spouse's needs.

If your children are grown and away, you will want to consider seriously and carefully whether you want them to come home. You are entitled to express your preference. They have the right to decide what they will do. You need to weigh the emotional benefits of their presence against the potential disruption in all of your lives. How can you keep yourself from feelings if you have to take of them too? Will you be loving and supportive to each other, or will old family conflicts flare up and cause additional pain?

One man thought twice before calling their son, away at college during exam week, to inform him that his mother had suffered a heart attack. Another cardiac spouse made the decision, with her fingers crossed, not to send for her two daughters, who were off at music camp. Still another knew instinctively that her thirty-year-old daughter wouldn't rest easy until she saw her father with "her own two eyes."

Some patients are adamant about not wanting anyone but you at the hospital. Some fathers don't want to "bother the children," or have them "see Dad this way." They would prefer the kids to come when they're out of the hospital and feeling less vulnerable at home. Others are comforted by having the whole family gathered round.

Director of Communications is the position you assume, as you handle the information clearinghouse. Your access to the patient makes you the obvious source of information for family and friends. Because you are closest to the situation, you are expected to relay messages and provide medical reports. Everyone means well and sends their love and best wishes. Their support is appreciated, but it's exhausting to repeat every detail of recovery each time someone calls. You wish you had a press secretary so the information could be passed more efficiently.

How can you think about everyone else's needs when you can barely get your own head on straight? You may be asked indirectly whether you think your husband will survive. You may not be prepared or willing to confront this question. Young children may ask directly, "Is my Daddy going to die?" is there a way to provide an honest and realistic answer and still manage to comfort your child. What is good counsel for your grown son, who is trying to make a decision about leaving his own family in another part of the country to be with you and his father?

You cannot always make wise decisions when you are dealing with the unknown. What if your mate doesn't survive? Would it be better or worse if the children were present? What are the psychological risks if they aren't there and their father dies? There are no easy answers. Good judgment is difficult when your mind is scattered and you are confused.

Don't let other people's urgency and fear pressure you. You may be too upset or exhausted to make any decisions, except for those that are absolutely critical. And remember that "I don't know" is a perfectly acceptable answer. *You're not responsible for knowing everything.* You can't predict the future.

What You Need to Know about Your Thinking

It usually takes time, sometimes as much as several months, for your mind to return to its normal level of functioning. Some cardiac spouses have chronic problems concentrating and remembering details, since they are still so preoccupied. One woman who was habitually a voracious reader, couldn't focus her attention long enough to follow magazine recipes for the first six months after her husband's heart attack. Another woman had to bring work home with her, because her shortened attention span caused her to fall behind on the job.

I was particularly unnerved by an incident that showed how distracted I was. One day, several weeks after

*Marsh's heart attack, I was driving home from work. When I
turned off the ignition, I was surprised to find myself in the
driveway of our old house. We hadn't lived there for over two
years. I must have been driving on "automatic pilot," or
maybe I unconsciously wanted to turn time back. In either
case, I felt scared by how disoriented I was. I wondered if it
was safe for me to drive. I even thought I might be going crazy.*

    Uncontrollable circular thinking is another symp-
tom that affects cardiac spouses. Like a broken record,
your mind goes over and over the events of the heart attack
or surgery. You may repeat the same stories, lose your train
of thought, or be totally unable to think about anything else.
You may find this repetitive thinking occurring for many
weeks into the recovery period.

    Another Phenomenon that is instinctively triggered
when people confront sudden and unexpected loss is a
mechanism called "life review."1 The most important events
of your life are quickly and vividly recalled, like they are
when you have a near miss while driving on the highway
and your whole life flashes by you before you've braked to
a halt. If you recall getting the news of your spouse's heart
attack, you may remember experiencing a partial life review. In less than a minute you mentally saw the highlights
of your whole marriage. While this was happening, you may
have momentarily lost track of time or been thoroughly
absorbed in another world. None of this means that you've
lost your mind. On the contrary, life review is a natural
process which prepares you to deal with loss.

    It is normal and healthy to relive your experience.
Your mind is trying to make sense of shocking and chaotic
events. The process of mental repetition brings order out of
chaos. Repeating the details of your experience aloud, you
clarify and deepen your understanding.

    While the urgent need to share you experience
diminishes over time, cardiac spouses exchange stories for
years with as much intensity as if the events had just

happened. Although many years have passed, I still get emotional while thinking and talking about Marsh's heart attacks. Be kind and patient with yourself. Be sure to give yourself as much time as you need. Meeting with other cardiac spouses will give you the opportunity to tell your story and listen long after friends and neighbors have lost interest. Sharing serves a purpose; perhaps it is even necessary if you are to integrate your experience and continue your personal growth.

Surviving the acute crisis doesn't automatically relieve the stresses and pressures that you know exist. A number of detailed responsibilities follow you home from the hospital. You must be attentive and alert to communicate with the doctor, supervise your mate's medications, and structure a new dietary plan. Beyond coping with daily tasks, you need your mind clear to make ongoing decisions and to confront the deeper meaning of the crisis.

Untangling the Web

Your thoughts and your feelings are closely intertwined. Anxiety makes your thinking less rational. And when you're not thinking rationally, your anxiety accelerates—a vicious cycle. In a crisis, powerful feelings wrap themselves around your mind like a blanket, suffocating you. No matter how hard you try to concentrate, you end up panicky and confused. Fears about the future paralyze you until you can't think. Even after you make a decision, your fear can stop you, freezing any action.

If you're blaming yourself for not being more organized and decisive—*stop*. It's very likely that your feelings are getting in the way. Whether you are seeking information, have an important decision to make, or need the solutions to more unanswered questions, the first step is to deal with your feelings. Acknowledging your feelings is important. If you know what you're feeling, you can calm down and begin to think logically.

Gathering information is a positive way to dispel anxiety. Most people cope better when they have the whole story. Without it, your imagination runs wild, creating scenarios far worse than reality. If you're like most cardiac spouses, you probably have a slew of unspoken, unaddressed, and unanswered questions. They may torment you when you are trying to sleep or pop up at odd times, catching you unaware. You may find them circling around and around in your head without any landing gear. First, organize your questions into a list. I strongly recommend keeping a pad of paper and a pencil handy, day and night. Write down any question that comes up. Or, you can ask your questions aloud to yourself or to someone willing to listen.

Once you have access to your questions, you can categorize them. Separate them into two groups: those that are unanswerable and those that have potential answers. For the time being, set aside the questions that don't have answers. Focus on questions to which there are answers in order to reduce you anxiety and empower yourself toward action. Using your mind will reassure you that you haven't lost it.

Next, divide your questions into two subgroups: informational questions and decision-making questions. Informational questions provide data about your mate's condition, prognosis, and the repercussions of his disease. With this information you will begin to see the truths of your situation. Some sample informational questions include:

What causes heart disease?
What are the newest medical treatments that may prolong
      my spouse's life?
How long will recovery take?
What life-style limitations can we anticipate?

When is it safe to resume sexual activity?

Obtaining information is an ongoing process. A trip to the library to borrow material about heart disease will provide you with some valuable information. So can attendance at lectures and participation in seminars for cardiac patients and their families. Not only will you get answers to your questions, but you may learn something that can directly improve your spouse's recovery. If you aren't accustomed to being persistent and assertive, this seeking out of information can be difficult but empowering. You may find yourself hesitant to ask strangers about highly personal things, but try not to let fear or embarrassment stop you from finding out what you need to know. Sources for information include:

American Heart Association National Center
7320 Greenville Avenue
Dallas, Texas 75231
(Use your phone book to locate your state office)

American Association of Cardiovascular
      and Pulmonary Rehabilitation
7611 Elmwood Avenue, Suite 201
Middleton, Wisconsin 53562
(608) 831-6989

Heartmates®
P.O. Box 16202
Minneapolis, Minnesota 55416

Cardiac Rehabilitation Programs at your local hospital, YMCA, or Jewish Community Center

Write to, call, or visit any of these organizations. What you learn will benefit you and your mate.

Mustering up courage to discuss sexual activity with your physician might turn out to be well worth your while. Steady your mind and seek answers to your questions. It will only increase your confidence in yourself as you cope with your crisis.

Decision-making questions have a different purpose from informational questions. They are geared to help you think about issues so you can make informed decisions. Some sample decision-making questions include:

How should I inform family members about a change in my
     spouse's condition?
Should my spouse go ahead with bypass surgery?
Should we plan a winter vacation in the sun?
What financial adaptations do we need to make?
What changes need I consider about my career or
     retirement?
What life-style changes should we make? Should I make?

Five Elements of Clear Thinking Before Making a Decision

Crisis is not an ideal time to make decisions. You feel especially vulnerable, unable to think clearly. And yet you are expected to make important decisions that just can't be postponed. It helps to approach the process in an organized fashion. I have broken down the process into five categories to make it simpler and less overwhelming. Consider each of these elements before you make a decision.

1. **Priority.** How important is the decision?
2. **Involving Others.** Is this a decision to be made alone or with others?
3. **Time.** How urgent is the decision?

4. **Action.** Is this an active or receptive decision?
5. **Purpose.** What is my purpose and goal?

1. WHAT'S THE PRIORITY

It is vital that you differentiate between big and little decisions. Your energy is limited, and you are more likely to spin your wheels unless you clarify the priorities. Once you decide that something is really significant., you can concentrate your attention and make a decision based on your assessment of all the possible consequences. If it's truly important, it deserves your most educated consideration. If it's not a high priority, you can let it wait.

Of course, when you are upset, fatigued, and confused, it isn't always obvious which decisions are critical or urgent. What you really need is perspective. Ask a trusted friend to look at your list of decisions; it might help you to see more clearly. I advise the following rule of thumb for assessing priorities: Judge a decision's importance by how much it concerns you. If making a medical decision is consistently on your mind, take care of it before moving on to other things. If life-style issues are most confusing, give them your attention. You also need to verify that your concerns are realistic. Sharing your list with someone who is compassionate but less involved can give you the opportunity to look at the issue in light of the bigger picture. Once you have arranged your decisions in order of priority, based on the intensity of your concern and a reality check, you can deal with them one at a time.

2. INVOLVING OTHERS

The next consideration is how to make a decision. Since you are the healthy one, it stands to reason that you should make the decisions. On the other hand, they directly affect your mate. Certain decisions may seem to trivial, a waste of his energy, and others so stressful as to place him at risk. Some cardiac spouses assume full responsibility, choosing to exclude their husbands, other family members, medical staff, or trusted friends who can offer suggestions and provide another perspective. This can be controlling and isolating; remember results of decisions often have an impact on the whole cardiac family.

In the best circumstances, you hope you are able to take other people's needs into consideration. Making decisions alone or cooperatively is a matter of individual style. In a crisis people usually fall back on what is most familiar, but that may not be the best prescription for the situation at hand. If you are a person who usually thinks and decides alone, you may want to consider the advantages of asking others for help. And if you are a person who tends to rely on others, you might consider thinking these decisions through on your own. Ultimately, you have the right to make decisions in whatever way works best for you.

3. THE ASPECT OF TIME

Timing is yet another serious element in decision making. There are decisions that need to be made instantaneously, and others in which there is plenty of time to plan. Maintaining a clear sense of time can be tricky. In a crisis, your sense of time becomes distorted. Time can seem to stretch out infinitely when you are waiting to hear how your spouse has come through bypass surgery. Or a long time can pass in the flash of a millisecond when you picture your years together before the cardiac crisis. When you are making a decision, it is important to differentiate urgency of the need for speed from adequate time to make the wisest decision.

Barely two months after Marsh's recovery from a second mild heart attack, his cardiologist suggested that he

*have an angiogram. His opinion afterward: no surgery indi-
cated; proceed with conservative treatment, including diet,
exercise, and medication.*

*Thoroughly frightened by two heart attacks, we de-
cided to seek a second opinion from a different cardiologist.
He advised the exact opposite, saying, "If I were you, I'd have
surgery as soon as possible." We were stunned! It had never
dawned on us that getting a second opinion would complicate our decision. We naively had expected it to verify that
Marsh's cardiologist was "right" and to reassure us because
we felt so vulnerable and powerless.*

*We had been hoping to increase our security. Instead,
our anxiety was multiplied.*

*Our purpose was clear. we were committed to doing
whatever would be best for Marsh's health. But what was
best? We struggled with the decision for a week, going over
the advantages and disadvantages in our minds.*

*We felt powerfully drawn toward a decision in favor
of surgery. We both wanted Marsh to live the active life of a
normal forty-five-year-old. If we chose surgery, we thought
our panic would diminish. and that somehow Marsh would
be safer. And it would feel as if we were doing something-
anything-to relieve the mounting tension.*

*But the disadvantages were obvious, too. Having just
gone through two recent recovery periods, surgery would
mean starting over a third time. It would take another three
to six months to rebuild Marsh's physical strength and
endurance. We knew that bypass surgery was no guarantee
that Marsh would not have a third heart attack or that he
would live a longer life.*

*Marsh's cardiologist gave us articles to read from the
highly respected New England Journal of Medicine which
corroborated his interpretation. He reminded us that time
was in our favor; cardiac research was rapidly developing
new technology that was less dangerous and more effective.
Since heart disease was progressive, it would be wise to save
surgery, an invasive, risky treatment, until it was necessary.
He assured us that if anything in Marsh's condition changed,
surgery would be seriously considered. From beginning to
end, our cardiologist was logical, informative, and respectful of every question we asked.*

*Finally, we decided. Marsh would go with the more
conservative treatment; he would not have bypass surgery.
Just reaching a decision helped to reduce our anxiety and*

stress. Eventually, Marsh stopped feeling like a time bomb about to explode. Because we had shared the decision-making process, we both felt unequivocally committed to Marsh's recovery plan. He reaffirmed his choice with his strong
commitment to regular exercise in a cardiac rehabilitation class. He took his medications regularly, and he assumed responsibility for moderating his diet.

Almost two years passed before circumstances changed radically. One morning Marsh awakened with severe chest pains that were only sporadically relieved by nitroglycerin. Walking the half block from the parking lot to his office left him short of breath. Urgency and fear returned to our lives. Our cardiologist scheduled an angiogram and surgery for the following day. Now our decision was urgent: Marsh's life was on the line. And again we were faced with a choice. This time the choice was to have bypass surgery. Although we were scared about the surgery and disappointed that it was necessary after all the changes Marsh had made, we were satisfied that it was the right choice.

4. ACTION AND INACTION

Most people consider decision making as exclusively active. To most of us, making a decision means taking a stand or doing something. In fact, decision making often involves acceptance and trust, and being receptive to someone else's judgment. As you accept the fact that there is nothing to be done, you actually have done something. A decision not to act, not to schedule bypass surgery after Marsh's heart attacks, was as much of a decision as choosing to do so two years later.

You must understand that any decision is simultaneously saying "yes" to something, and "no" to something else. Every "yes" is also "no"! We generally ignore what needs a "no," because it may be uncomfortable or unpleasant. Your decision to establish a heart-healthy diet requires you to say "no" to fatty meats and salty soups.

Whether your decision requires action or maintenance of the status quo, try to be positively involved in the process. This means initiating action when it is appropriate and choosing to remain still when that will be most beneficial.

Accepting inaction in the face of danger requires courage and faith. There's little in life that is demanding than simply waiting and being receptive to what comes.

5. ESTABLISHING GOALS

Finally, you'll need to explore your underlying purpose so you can define your goals— it's a prerequisite to good decision making. To establish purpose, you will have to ask the question, "why?" Struggling with that "why?" may not yield a specific answer, but it will help you pinpoint and solidify your goals. Your purpose might be general, like expressing the love that you feel for your spouse, or specific, like understanding and supporting a new dietary regimen. Your purpose forms the natural foundation for the decisions want to make.

Pamela, a talented and respected counselor, became a cardiac spouse just after her fiftieth birthday. About six months after her husband's heart attack, she asked me to help her with a career decision. Pamela and Christopher's financial situation was secure. He had a solid offer to sell his small business, and decided, at age fifty-three, to retire early.

Until Chris' heart attack, their marriage had been satisfying, but secondary. With two full-time careers and no children, they were both accustomed to being independent and going their own ways. Christopher's illness brought them closer together. Pamela discovered that her husband meant more to her than she had ever thought. Confronted with the possibility of losing him, she realized that she wanted to make their relationship a higher priority in her life.

Pamela's goal was to reorganize her time so that it matched her new values. She tried to weigh the pros and cons of keeping or giving up her career. Retiring would mean that she and Chris would have more time together. They would be able to relax, spend time quietly at their cabin, and escape the stress of city life.

On the surface, it seemed like a perfect solution. Her family had never been supportive of her need for a career; it had always been a disappointment to them that Pamela hadn't chosen to be a housewife and mother. On the other hand, her work was a big part of what made her feel valued. Having her own earned income, although it was much smaller than Chris', enhanced her feelings of independence and provided a sense of maturity that parenthood may otherwise have given her. And without her job, she felt as if she would be giving up the only thing that she could really call her own.

As she reexamined her priorities, Pamela realized how much she valued her marriage and her career. Both emerged as powerful rivals for top of her list of priorities, so she decided to choose a workable, meaningful compromise. She elected to see clients only on Tuesdays, Wednesdays, and Thursdays, an arrangement that freed up the rest of her week to spend with Chris. Staying in touch with her original goal helped Pamela turn an "either/or" decision into a "both/and" opportunity.

Staying in touch with your purpose while you act is difficult, particularly during the acute phase of the cardiac crisis, and even as you reorient your life during recovery. The cardiac crisis often opens to question old values you have taken for granted, while not necessarily offering answers. Major decisions require investigation and understanding followed by realignment of your actions with your carefully considered values. Taking time to think about your decisions can keep you connected to the purpose behind your actions. And committing them to paper, as you write what you feel, can help you stay on track. Here is a Heartmates® Guide for you to use as you work through the process of decision making.

HEARTMATES® GUIDE FOR DECISION MAKING

1. What is the decision facing me? (State it as clearly as possible.)
2. What is my purpose for making this decision?
3. What options open to me would help me achieve my purpose? (List all options you can think of, including those you know you would not ultimately chose.)
4. What are the positives and negatives (the costs) of each of these options? What can I predict as the result or consequence of each option? To me? To my spouse? To our family? To others?
5. What feelings do I have as I consider this decision?
6. Are there things I need to know, to learn about, before I can think through this decision? (How can I get the information I need?)
7. Once you have considered these questions, make your decision, and commit it to writing: "I have decided to..."; or "I choose to..."
8. How do I feel about having made this decision? (Is ambivalence or another feeling getting in the way of my acting on my choice?)
9. Don't avoid necessary decisions. Not deciding is a decision.
10. Remember your original purpose as you act on your decision. (Use this guide to keep you connected to your goals.)
11. Celebrate your success!

Considering the Deeper Questions

The cardiac crisis brings you face to face with how much control you have. Sometimes, no matter how well informed or decisive you are, there are areas over which you have little or no authority. You can't make heart disease disappear; you can't change what has already happened to you and your mate because of heart disease. You can't even change how you feel about it. Your power is limited to choosing what your attitude will be about what is happening. You can be in charge of the way you will accept and adapt to a new reality, a new life.

Living with unanswerable questions is painful. It is a rare and unusual individual who would choose uncertainty over security. But accepting your powerlessness also has its rewards.

Your day-to-day life has been ruptured by cardiac crisis. All your perceptions are altered. The result can be an awakening to a new level of thinking, deeper than your prevailing habit permits. You may experience it as a sense that something is different. You may have a momentary flash that "life is not forever" or that "this relationship is precious." Many cardiac spouses do not recognize these flashes, because the everyday mind is so insistent and demanding. Those who have this revelation describe it as a whisper rising in the rare moments when the mind calms down.

The whisper directs the cardiac spouse to the deeper questions that are an integral, though often buried, part of the cardiac crisis. These questions invite you to explore issues beyond medications, diets, and daily routines. They provoke serious thoughts about mortality, purpose, and the meaning of life. They ask you to look at yourself in relation to the larger world, to other cardiac spouses, to others in pain, and to all others on the planet.

The everyday part of the mind races clamorously, scrambling for concrete answers; it loves cholesterol levels and milligrams, the countable and the knowable. The whispering question doesn't seek the right answer; it only needs permission to be heard. Simply contemplating issues and struggling to understand questions will enable you to grow emotionally.

Sure, it's easier to stay involved with the practical questions because the unknown is so disconcerting. Many cardiac spouses may have conscientiously avoided such questions since childhood or adolescence. Others have outgrown the answers they accepted then, but haven't had the occasion to reexamine them until now. Still others may be disillusioned by the idealistic answers of youth. It is natural to push nagging questions away by saying, "None of this really matters" or "I haven't got time to think about this, because I have to take care of the everyday tasks that fill my life" or, like Scarlett O'Hara, promise yourself to think about it tomorrow.

I propose that recovery is an ideal time to ponder the realm of meaning and purpose. The cardiac crisis has made you vulnerable, and you are more likely to see the gravity of those deeper questions about the meaning and quality of life. The protection of normal, daily life and the illusions of being powerful and in full control over your life are broken down, so that the whisper can be heard.

Should you choose to respond, make sure to give yourself some regular quiet time. Find a place where you can think undisturbed; go for a walk, take a long, hot bath, or sit in your favorite easy chair. Start a diary or a journal to keep an ongoing record of your experience, for later reflection. Or pursue your thoughts and questions by sharing them with a trusted friend. There is no "right" way to ponder the deeper questions. Whatever your individual style is, take advantage of the opportunity.

SOME THOUGHTS ON THINKING

- Limited concentration and inability to focus are normal responses to a cardiac crisis.
- Normal thinking patterns return more slowly than feelings.
- Reviewing the events of your cardiac story is a natural and healing mental response.
- Repetition transforms chaos and confusion into a sense of order and meaning.
- Recognizing feelings is a first step to untangling thoughts.
- Sharing thoughts can give you another's perspective and a valuable reality check.
- Postpone unnecessary decision making whenever possible, until you have control over your thinking.
- The everyday, rational part of your mind is an important resource in decision making.
- The quiet, abstract part of your mind connects you to questions of meaning and to your internal wisdom.

Shifting Responsibility

*B*efore the cardiac crisis, you had a busy, active life. You probably weren't looking for any extra work or stress. Whether at home, in your marriage, or in your career, you could handle the daily demands of your life.

But from the moment your mate became a cardiac patient, your responsibilities changed. Regardless of what the division of labor had been prior to the cardiac event, you now find yourself saddled with both your mate's and your own shares.

In the acute stage of the crisis, your responsibilities simply snowballed. Suddenly, you were in charge of medical decisions, financial arrangements, and the emotional needs of your family. At the most extreme, your mate was bedridden, perhaps unable to speak. His only responsibility was to rest so that his heart would heal. You were responsible for everything else.

The dramatic switch in responsibility is intensified because you are in crisis. Your anxiety is heightened and even simple decisions seem overwhelming. Normal demands seem heavier and less manageable. And the crisis creates new jobs and still more responsibilities as you must inform family and friends, and run the household single-handedly.

Once your mate returns home, your hands are full in other ways. Because economic considerations make hospital stays shorter, you end up having to give your husband semi-skilled nursing care. Your spouse's physical activity is limited, and he still spends much of his time in bed. The majority of your time is spent preparing and serving meals, changing bedding, and monitoring medications.

It's also incumbent on you to make sure that friends and family don't overstay their visits. You feel it's up to you to make sure that your mate doesn't get overly taxed or exhausted. And, despite your own fatigue, you may feel obligated to play hostess by taking reservations for visiting hours, serving coffee and sweets, and cleaning up after the guests are gone.

Entertaining only adds to your stress when you are coping with a crisis. Some visitors are a source of comfort, and you welcome them with open arms, but others are more of a hindrance than a help. Some guests stop by, pay attention to the patient, eat a bite, and disappear (sort of life doting grandparents who leave before the diapers have to be changed). Other visitors arrive with food, flowers, and gifts of love and support.

This is not the time for you to put other people's needs first. You have stretched yourself to the your physical and emotional limits. Kudos of appreciation for you are in order. Assuming a cardiac spouse's responsibilities deserves respect and recognition from you, your mate, and others. And yet you may be tempted to tolerate inconvenient or insensitive visitors out of politeness. You may feel guilty turning away guests who might cheer up your mate. But this is your home, too. If you can, try to overcome your feelings of obligation. If you feel you have to stand on ceremony with some people, ask them to visit at a later date.

Once you enter the recovery phase, new and different responsibilities emerge. If your spouse has had to face early retirement, you may be financially pressured and have to become the sole breadwinner. Running back and forth between your job and home adds more anxiety and stress.

Cardiac patients are often depressed, and by default they leave the majority of daily responsibilities to you. Even if your mate is recovering relatively smoothly, you might still spend hours catering heart-healthy meals or running to the pharmacy. Or, perhaps months down the road, you find yourself stuck, unable to stop constantly "baby-sitting" your mate.

Shifting responsibility is one of the most complex issues you face. On the surface, the chose seems obvious: Your mate needs help, so its natural for you to assume the responsibility. And the fact that he's depending on you makes you want to rise to the occasion.

Because of the unexpected and sudden onset of the cardiac crisis, you simply take on whatever needs to be done. You may believe that you have no choice and that loving your spouse means pickling up all the slack.

How much responsibility you take on can be measures quite easily. Look at how you spend your time. However, understanding you patterns of responsibility, and how much you and your mate depend on each other, is more complicated. Patterns that take years to develop become firmly entrenched in your relationship. Caring for your sick spouse has either cemented existing patterns, or created entirely new ones.

You may or may not be aware of how your responsibilities have changed. Each new task that you have added to your repertoire may have been a conscious choice. Or you may have gradually added more and more without being aware of it. You feel as if all your existing responsibilities are equally important and you can't alter them. But before you can consider any future action, you need to aware of how your responsibilities have *already* changed.

Answer the following questions to delineate your changing responsibilities. Begin by evaluating your "normal" (pre-cardiac crisis) responsibilities. Then, look at your new responsibilities.

HEARTMATES® RESPONSIBILITY QUESTIONNAIRE

Before the cardiac crisis:

1. Which spouse took more responsibility in each of the following areas:

_____ earning a living
_____ handling the family finances
_____ meals
_____ housework
_____ yard work
_____ parenting your children
_____ caring for aging parents
_____ social and recreational activities
_____ your relationship with each other
_____ spiritual life

2. In what ways was your spouse dependent on you?
3. In what ways were you dependent on your spouse?
4. Have the two you become more or less dependent on each other throughout the life of your relationship?
5. Did you consider yourself:

_____ independent
_____ too independent

_____ dependent
_____ too dependent
_____ interdependent
_____ responsible
_____ overresponsible
_____ underresponsible

Since the cardiac crisis:

1. What responsibilities are different now?
   What do you do now that's different?
   How do you feel about your new responsibilities?
2. List ways in which you are more dependent on your spouse now.
3. List ways in which you are less dependent on your spouse now.
4. In what ways is your spouse more dependent on you now?
5. In what ways is your spouse more independent from you now?

Identifying and understanding changes in responsibility earmarks the beginning of *your* recovery. Whether you have taken on more responsibility consciously or as a matter of course, these new patterns form the foundation of your relationship. Habits establish themselves quickly. Temporary emergency measures quickly evolve into a permanent change in division of labor.

Some cardiac spouses thrive on extra pressure and responsibility. If you're the kind of person who's prone to take care of your mate or if you take pride in being at your best in an emergency, you might welcome the opportunity to take charge. Other spouses feel weary, resentful, and yearn for less pressure and more peace. Any and all of these responses are fine. You just need to know what's actually going on so that you can judge the progress of your recovery and appraise your relationship.

Responsibility and Love

It is natural and appropriate to assume more responsibility during a cardiac crisis. There is nothing more disturbing than seeing someone you love helpless and suffering. You want to do anything and everything you can to help. Cardiac spouses should be awarded a "purple heart for bravery" for just standing by. Your genuine love and concern for your spouse is expressed when you take charge in a loving and compassionate way.

After Marsh's bypass surgery, he was moved into the intensive care unit. I was thoroughly unprepared for what I witnessed when I first saw him there. Under the huge overhead heating lamp, and attached to several strange-sounding machines and the respirator, Marsh looked like an alien from outer space. He lay very still and his skin felt cold and stiff. He was barely awake, and was receiving morphine for pain.

Marsh had been invaded—to his very core. A half dozed tubes he could not control led in and out of his body. Even his hose and throat had tubes running into them, making it impossible for him to speak. He had no way to say, "Please scratch my nose, it itches." He had no way to let me know that his lips were dry, and that he would appreciate something cool and wet. He had no way to express his fear, anger, or hurt. He had no way to celebrate the fact that he was alive.

I felt immense compassion for him. I chose to be Marsh's protection, his shield. I committed myself to being the buffer between his total vulnerability and the outside world.

We quickly devised a system so that he could communicate. He would write out his questions or statements, tracing one letter at a time with his finger on the sheet at his side. I read his tracing aloud, and when I was correct, he would move on. If not, he would indicate my mistake by raising his index finger, and repeat the letter again. It was a slow process. Sometimes he would forget in the middle of spelling a word and slide into a morphine snooze. (Magic slates or small dry-erase boards and markers should be standard equipment in cardiac care units.)

The first question I Marsh traced on the sheet was, "What time is it?" I looked at my watch and told him it was 4:30. He reacted by becoming very upset. His hand returned to the sheet, and he began tracing again. "W-H-A-T D-A-Y? "Through this primitive communication, I began to understand how lost, how helpless, how vulnerable Marsh was. He didn't even know what day it was or how long he had been there. Although it had been a long and difficult day for me too, I vowed to stand there until I couldn't stand anymore, to do what I could for this man I loved so much.

Later the same evening one of the monitoring machines made a new noise, beeping a different message than before. I was asked to step out of the unit, and when I returned Marsh seemed very agitated. Back to the sheet and the letter tracing. One letter at a time, but I got the picture. Marsh had tried to ask the nurse why the machine was making the noise. Her response: "Don't worry about it; you're doing fine." If she had intended to reassure Marsh, she had succeeded in accomplishing the opposite. Being patronized only aggravated his concern.

When the nurse returned, I asked about the sound. She repeated what she'd said to Marsh. I said that I wanted to know. She explained that the machine was reporting a malfunction. Within minutes, the machine was replaced with another that beeped like a familiar friend.

I was Marsh's shield, his voice, and his protection. It was necessary . . . and satisfying. The next morning brought a change. The tubes were removed from his throat, and he was able to speak for himself.

As soon as Marsh could talk, my speaking for him grew insulting. When patients are just out of surgery, or have just suffered a heart attack, they require total care, as do newborn children. But just as children gradually become more independent, cardiac patients rapidly advance from total vulnerability to a level where they are able to take care of themselves. A parent who takes too much responsibility fosters dependence, and handicaps rather than helps a child. The same is true of cardiac spouses. At each stage of recovery, it's crucial for you to determine what your mate can and can't handle, relinquishing your responsibility accordingly.

You might be genuinely pleased to see your mate gradually taking care of his own needs. His increased involvement is a positive sign of recovery. Or you might experience some ambivalence. Just as some parents find it hard to let go, you might feel hesitant about stepping back and letting your spouse fend for himself.

Supporting your mate's recovery means noticing and encouraging his efforts toward independence. While you are understandably worried that he might do too much and have a relapse, do not allow your fear to stand in the way of his recovery. After witnessing your spouse's utter helplessness in the hospital, how can you help being overly protective? A cardiac spouse will have some trouble shifting gears and discovering how much her mate can realistically handle. Sometimes this causes a serious problem. One cardiac spouse insisted on spoon-feeding her husband even though he had been eating without assistance since the first day after surgery. Another man imposed mandatory rest periods, even when his wife wasn't tired.

Medical warnings to avoid stress are often misunderstood. Cardiac spouses may "take over" to protect their mates from the danger of undue stress. A most extreme example is the cardiac spouse who forbade her husband to watch television news. Each morning she clipped out all the newspaper articles she thought were too stressful for him to read.

Recovery is an emotional as well as a physical process. Just as you need to continually reassess your idea of your mate's physical progress, you need to review your image of him as a patient. As he becomes stronger, you have to be willing to change your image of yourself, from heroine to helpmate. You must not do everything, only your appropriate share.

If you're afraid to stop overprotecting your mate, remember that heart patients are weaned from total care in a graduated, step-by-step plan by the hospital nursing staff. You can feel confident that he is well enough to function without round-the-clock care and can begin doing things for himself.

Maintaining the role of patient or "victim" over the long haul is emotionally destructive and will slow you mate's physical recovery. Encouraging your spouse to remain helpless isn't healthy for either of you. Both of you are in a period of recovery. While your efforts to help are clearly motivated by caring and concern, taking on too much responsibility may ultimately backfire, trapping you into doing more than you should. A combination of rest and some responsibility is the best way for your mate to regain strength and confidence. And your recovery also depends on a shifting balance of power and responsibility.

Responsibility and Fear

The right responsibility is supportive and loving. However, in a cardiac crisis there is the risk of assuming too much responsibility. In this context, "right" responsibility means basing your actions on an accurate perception of reality. For example, calling the rescue squad when your mate is having unremitting chest pain is perfectly appropriate. However, calling the doctor every time your spouse looks pale is a sign of over responsibility. Taking on more responsibility than is actually warranted is certainly a sign that fear is making you overreact.

Fear is the number one cause of overresponsibility. Feelings are powerful and fear is no exception. The fear you experience may be out of proportion to the present situation—like when you're convinced that your mate is on the verge of another heart attack, even though the physician just prescribed more physical activity and less medication.

Cardiac spouses entertain a wide range of exaggerated fears, from losing sleep over one salty pretzel to fantasizing divorce based on an angry outburst.

Your fears may go back to an earlier time when you felt as though you were in danger. When fear is triggered, the feeling is intensified by memories of childhood—of a time when you were more helpless and dependent. Nearly losing your mate could summon those feelings once again.

Intense fear coupled with the all consuming sense of responsibility produces an awesome burden, not at all unlike bringing your first newborn home from the hospital. Everything revolves around the baby's schedule and demands. When you're not busy caring for your baby, you worry if he or she is okay. Remember listening intently for the sounds indicating that the baby was still alive after a nap or a night's sleep?

Obviously, your mate is not a totally helpless infant. And you are not totally helpless as far as coping with your fear of losing your mate is concerned. Yet when the fear escalates, you might respond by acting overly responsible, staying awake all night to check your mate's breathing, or waking him up to ask him if he took his medications.

Listening for your partner's breathing is a perfectly normal reaction after all you've been through. But sacrificing your sleep in order to be the permanent night nurse is a sign of deeper, perhaps unfounded fears.

Survival Fears

If you're like most cardiac spouses, your worst fear is that your mate will die and you will be left alone. Beneath this is the deepest dread: Can you survive that loss? If he dies, how will you go on?

How terrifying to consider the possibility of losing your mate! You may even believe that you can't live without him. But if you search within yourself, you know that you will survive. It may be difficult, painful, and very lonely, but few people actually die of a broken heart. I don't advocate obsession with morbid scenarios. However, you must face your worst fear and believe that you will come out safely on the other side.

Human beings have defense mechanisms to protect them from coping directly with such enormous threats. You are probably unaware that of the extent of your terror, on a day-to-day basis. The human mechanism devises ways to function even in the face of extreme fear. In order to go about your daily life, you may ignore, rationalize, or deny your fear. But whether or not you're consciously aware of it, your fear manifests itself in a number of ways in your relationship.

The heart-to-heart bond between you and your mate becomes a conduit for unvoiced fears. While you each have unique fears, they reinforce and feed each other's. You may be anxious about your mate coming home from the hospital, doubting your ability to provide adequate care. He senses your insecurity and begins to question whether he's well enough to leave. Once home, you try to limit your spouse's activities so he won't "overdo." Before you know it he's checking his pulse several times a day and expects you to coddle him, convinced that he'd better not strain himself. One spouse, afraid for her husband to leave the security of home, avoided all social activities. She even turned down invitations to their children's homes for Sunday dinner.

Fear makes loving couples turn away from much-needed physical affection. It's typical for cardiac couples to wrongly assume that sexual intercourse is too strenuous to be risked. Many couples pull back without discussing it, each believing that he or she is protecting the other. Your recovering spouse may feel afraid of disappointing you by having less vitality or strength. And after everything you've been told about not "exciting" the patient, it's not easy to relax and enjoy. But physical intimacy can comfort and reassure you. Loss of intimacy does not diminish fear; it may even raise it.

Too Much Dependence

Heart patients have been known to express fear by acting overly dependent on their mates. What about the patient who wants his spouse to be the only visitor at the hospital? Without even telling her why, he expects his wife to sit in a bedside vigil all day, with no relief from any other visitors. And this behavior may continue once the patient is home. John, an extremely busy account executive with a television station, took off three weeks while his wife had bypass surgery. Well on her way to recovery, his wife continued to fabricate reasons to keep John home from work, and berated him whenever he left the house. Another spouse, Corrine, gave her husband a bell to ring when he needed her so she would be free to move around inside their house. Yet another spouse's frightened husband wouldn't grant her five minutes to do a load of laundry in the basement unless a close relative was nearby. Imagine her frustration, being a prisoner in her own home. In such situations, how can you tell where you end and your spouse begins?

Cardiac patients are naturally preoccupied with their symptoms and emotions. Your mate might cope with his feelings by exhibiting sullen, vociferous, or extremely demanding behavior in a desperate effort to regain control of his life. He may start acting like a prima donna, expecting you to wait on him hand and foot. And you may react by becoming even more focused on your spouse, lavishing extra attention on him, further adapting your lifestyle to his.

There are a number of areas in which you might assume overresponsibility in a sincere but misguided effort to appease your spouse. You could put yourself in charge of risk factor control, carefully investigating ingredients in foods, or becoming an outspoken advocate of nonsmoking. Some cardiac spouses take on the role of peacemaker and censor all communication among family members in an effort to keep the household stress-free. Others become increasingly isolated as they build a life-style centered around their mate's needs instead of their own.

These examples of overdependency remind me of symptoms of addiction. The difference here is that the addiction is to a spouse rather than to a chemical. An addict is a person whose well-being depends on an external source of support and security.1 You and your mate may be unwittingly involved in an addictive relationship. He needs you to take care of him, and your identity is dependent on providing his care. The longer this cycle continues, the harder it is to break.

My fear that Marsh would die and leave me led to overresponsible behavior that strained our relationship.

Once he was home from the hospital I felt so afraid, so powerless to keep him alive, that I endowed his pills with that power. If he just took every pill, on time, everything would be okay. He would recover. He wouldn't have another heart attack. He wouldn't die.

I reminded him regularly about his medications. It became a routine part of my day to check that he'd taken his pills at the prescribed hour. The fact that he lived through each day was proof that my reminders were working. It never occurred to me that I was interfering. It never crossed my mind that he heard anything but my concern. I never imagined that he resented my questions.

Once day, after listening to me go through my litany, my dear friend Shirley said, "He's a grown man, perfectly capable of monitoring his own medications. Stop nagging. It must be driving him crazy." I was so surprised. I hadn't heard myself nag. I thanked Shirley and went home to undo what by then had become an ingrained responsibility. It was excruciating for several days, like withdrawal from an addiction. It took all my energy to keep quiet, to keep from saying, "have you taken your pills?"

One morning I came across Marsh's pill box next to the bathroom sink. He had already left for his cardiac rehabilitation class and wouldn't return home until evening. I stood there, paralyzed, wondering whether I should take his pills to him at his class or drive downtown and deliver them to his office. For a brief moment, I fantasized Marsh on the verge of another heart attack. Surely if anything happened it would be my fault. Then I saw how silly that was. I said to myself, "He can take care of himself; it isn't my responsibility." And suddenly the spell was broken. I was free!

I beat the meds, but the real issue was bigger: to break the pattern of dependency that had deepened with Marsh's illness. I needed to deal with my fear, so that we could have an equal relationship, based on mutual dignity and respect.

That night, when Marsh came home, he asked me if I'd noticed that he'd forgotten his pills. I acknowledged seeing the box near the sink, and he said, "It's a good thing I had brought an extra day's dosage to keep in my desk drawer at the office." Marsh can take care of himself; he can handle the responsibility. I had been overreacting.

When you let your fear get the best of you it can have serious, long-term consequences. Once an isolated type of behavior becomes a habit, it is difficult to change. Recovery doesn't happen overnight or without effort. You must continue to face your fears and look at your actions.

Flexibility

"Right responsibility" also requires flexibility. In some cases, your mate may remain so incapacitated that you actually need to handle most of the responsibilities. If you are in this position, then the first step is to assess the situation. How much is your mate able to do without your help? What responsibilities are urgent, and which can be set aside? What are the tasks that only you can take care of, and

which are the responsibilities that can be shared by friends, relatives, or service providers? The keys to sorting out appropriate responsibility are: assessment, setting priorities, and flexibility.

One cardiac spouse, Rita, described her struggle with right and overresponsibility as a back-and-forth affair. Steve's first heart attack occurred twelve years ago. Just as he was getting back on his feet, he had a second heart attack. Recovery was slow, but Rita gradually resumed her own life, feeling less responsible for Steve's physical care.

Two years ago, Steve's condition deteriorated dramatically. After a third heart attack and congestive heart failure, he is now often mentally confused and requires constant monitoring. Through no fault of her own, Rita is back to doling out medications and assuming responsibility for Steve's physical well-being. She is hungry for her freedom and anxious to give up the role of nurse. Their one ray of hope is that Steve is currently a heart transplant candidate. In the meantime, Rita's responsibilities continue to shift from day to day.

It's natural to feel resentful when you have to assume an inordinate amount of responsibility, especially over a long period of time. You may feel sad or angry about the time and energy consumed in doing more than your share. And rightfully so. If your mate's condition requires you to take on greater long term responsibilities, allow yourself to feel the weight of the burden. Pretending to be Superwoman or grumbling under your breath won't help.

Wherever your mate is in the recovery process, you will need to keep reevaluating the situation. By combining flexibility with shared decision making, shifting responsibilities can be a positive part of your relationship.

This Heartmates® comparative checklist will help you to identify the difference between right responsibility and overresponsibility:

Right Responsibility	Overresponsibility
Based on reality	An overreaction
Makes you feel calm	Makes you feel panicky
Well thought out	Urgent
Planned	Reckless
Comes from confidence	Motivated by fear
Allows for flexibility	Rigid and uncompromising

The Stress Syndrome

Stress as a risk factor is one of the most misunderstood myths and mysteries of heart disease today. The word alone can send chills of terror up and down your spine. Early in the cardiac crisis, you're given the message "Don't stress the patient. "The warning is often interpreted as an injunction against sharing worries, concerns, and fears. You stifle your feelings, thinking that you are protecting your mate from stress. You may even take on your mate's worries, trying to lower his stress load by increasing your own.

Your mate is equally sensitive to the stress myth. Stress is one of the most loosely used and least understood words in the English language. Despite the lack of a widely accepted definition of stress, it is universally terrifying to heart patients.

Cardiac patients sometimes use "stress" as an excuse to avoid uncomfortable situations. It isn't unusual to hear a cardiac patient blame or threaten a spouse with some variation of the statement, "Don't raise your voice, you'll make me have another heart attack."

The term "stress" is used generically by many cardiac spouses as well. "I need help coping with stress" is really a call for help in dealing with uncomfortable feelings or for finding appropriate avenues of expression or relief. Physical outlets that help people relax are often termed "stress reducers." Running, or any type of exercise, therapeutic message, and warm baths are activities recommended to help the cardiac spouse reduce stress.

Dr. Robert Eliot's attempts to solve the mysteries of stress and its relationship to heart disease have been inconclusive. He maintains that while everyone of us knows, or thinks he knows, what stress is, each person experiences stress in a highly individual way.[2]

Another problem in defining stress is that it affects different people in different ways. Four weeks after her heart attack, Julie felt frustrated because her doctor hadn't given her permission to drive her car. It was stressful to depend on someone else to chauffeur her around. But the thought of driving by herself also made her anxious. She was reluctant to ask her doctor when she could resume driving, fearful that his answer would verify her worst fear: a permanent life-style of severely limited freedom and mobility.

Dr. Hans Selye's definitive book[3] considers the question of whether stress factors in the environment actually produce harmful effects. His findings reinforce the idea that stress is a necessary part of a person's life.

What stress is and how it works to our benefit or harm is not yet clear. Despite this, cardiac recovery decisions are often based on the myths. When physicians or cardiac patients make long-range decisions based on an assessment of stress level, they are dealing with a complex subject, with largely unknown consequences.

The notion that a stress-free life is a more meaningful or qualitatively better life is another myth. Eliminating stress from a cardiac patient's life is impossible. And creating and living in a controlled environment, totally devoid of stimulus or conflict, makes for a boring and meaningless existence. A certain amount of stress is necessary to remain vital. Dr. Selye contends that "Life without stress is death."

Before his heart attack Paul was a minister for twenty-five years. On the advice of his physician, he didn't return to his vocation, believing it was too psychologically stressful. He had become increasingly depressed and apathetic, wandering around the house like a captain without a ship. Between Nancy's income from her work as a medical technician and a pension Paul receives from the national office of their church, they are able to make ends meet. But that doesn't resolve the psychological damage to Paul, who has withdrawn his contribution to his community.

Who can say which is more stressful: to practice ministry, feeling needed and helpful, but heavily stressed by the demanding nature of his job, or to be a depressed pensioner, whose life stress is minimal? What are the consequences of Nancy reversing roles to become the major breadwinner and Paul being stripped of his life's work?

I believe there is not enough evidence available yet to make good recommendations about stress and its effects on cardiac patients and spouses.

The setting of physical limitations is a different and separate issue. A "stress test" determines a safe level of physical activity, and should be heeded as a guide for healthy levels of physical exertion. When a patient's work is physical in nature, stress test results may indicate necessary reductions in work. They also serve an important role in medical diagnosis and provide progress reports for the patient.

What about the stress that already exists at home? Both of you may be pointing fingers at each other, blaming the patient's rising blood pressure on each other's bad habits.

The condition of your marital relationship may add stress to an already volatile situation. The family is a complex system, made more vulnerable by today's social changes and fast pace. In a crisis, each of you is more likely to be impatient and intolerant. Fear and anxiety cause you to be more irritable so that things you used to be able to accept and ignore suddenly seem like a big deal. Try not to judge the quality of your marriage in the midst of a crisis. It wasn't perfect before, why should all the problems magically disappear now?

If you are lucky, your marriage is a support system and a haven. Probably, though, there are times when it is a source of comfort and other times when being with each other intensifies the stress. Even if it seems as if your marriage is the main source of stress in your life, keep in mind that the familiarity and continuity it provides is an important anchor during what would otherwise be a chaotic period. And remember: This is a time to be especially gentle and understanding with each other.

From Caring to Caretaking

A great deal of your time and energy is devoted to looking after the needs of your recovering mate. One reason that you've taken on so much responsibility is because you care. But that's not the only reason. There is "caretaking." Just as there is a distinction between right responsibility and overresponsibility, caring and caretaking are two different things.

Helplessness is the primary feeling behind caretaking behavior. When you see your spouse vulnerable or in pain, you feel helpless. You wish that you could do something to fix it. Since there is nothing you can do to change the reality of your mate's heart disease, you compensate for your feelings by taking control.

Consider the cardiac spouse whose mate refuses to quit smoking. Everyone knows that smoking is high on the list of risk factors for heart disease. Each cigarette adds to your growing fear of losing your mate. You feel the pain and sadness that goes with watching your spouse self-destruct. You may nag, cajole, beg, even get angry and accusatory to try to get him to quit. Nothing works.

In fact, *you are helpless!* Attempting to control the uncontrollable inevitably leads to an image of yourself as a failure.

Women in our culture learn early to be caretakers. Beginning at a young age, girls are rewarded for being sensitive to other people's feelings; by maturity they may be unable to recognize their own. When asked, many adult women find it impossible to know or say what *they* need. Consequently, their needs are suppressed or denied.

As much as women today may be resentful or rebellious about being caretakers, we tend to fall into this familiar role when we are in crisis. Being a caretaker provides the illusion of control, masks helplessness, and keeps us from getting our own needs met.

Your image of yourself also contributes to your tendency to be a caretaker. The stereotype of the "good woman" or the "little woman" is a portrait of a gentle, sweet, even-tempered, and, inherently, long-suffering woman. Many women have been conditioned to strive for this ideal. Many cardiac spouses struggle to maintain such a picture of themselves, even during a crisis. Everything is at risk, and the only tools the "good woman" has at hand are sweetness and a willingness to suffer for "her man." She doesn't recognize her own feelings. She doesn't know she has needs or that in order for her to recover from her crisis she needs to take care of herself. She has been granted no permission to express her resentment about having to care for a mate who may not be caring for himself. Or worse, she may be caring for a mate who is only caring about himself.

If you take responsibility for your mate's feelings, activities, and his life, he will become dependent and you will become resentful. The "good woman" continues to maintain a sweetness that tastes bitter, and caretaking that has lost its foundation of caring.

It is a commonly held premise that the heart patient's recovery is in the hands of his spouse. *It isn't!* However irrational, you may feel personally responsible for your mate's health, recovery, and even his life. But you're not! *You didn't cause his heart disease, and you can't cure it.*

Expressing your caring, rather than caretaking your mate, requires a delicate balance. No one can make another person change. You are helpless to do anything that can make your spouse take his illness seriously. Sometimes cardiac spouses use blame or shame in an effort to coerce their mates to quit smoking, eat carefully, take medications religiously, exercise regularly, and eliminate unnecessary stress. Many cardiac patients are admitted "workaholics" and may strongly resist changing or limiting their careers in response to their heart condition.

Your caretaking may be in direct proportion to your husband's denial. The more he pushes himself, the more you nag him to slow down. If he makes a joke about eating prime rib, you counter with a lecture on the evils of cholesterol. You tend to interpret anything less than perfection and instant reversal of decades-long habit as denial or irresponsibility. If his attitude reflects a lack of concern for his condition, you double your efforts, and exhaust yourself on his behalf.

The same is true when it comes to feelings. In our culture it is more acceptable for women to have and express feelings than it is for men. Up to now, heart disease has been principally a male disease. It is customary for male heart patients to ignore or deny their feelings of anger or sadness. Men also have learned to mask their fear with bravado. Over many years, you and your mate's emotions have become so intertwined, that you may unconsciously take on his unexpressed feelings.

At one time or another, you've probably said, "I'm carrying the weight of the world on my shoulders," or "I'm worrying for both of us." There's real danger in assuming your mate's feelings. You can't carry the burden without exacting a cost to yourself. The consequence is your sense of failure, depression, even despair. Your genuine concern and desire to protect your mate will ultimately backfire, resulting in the opposite effect. If your mate doesn't have to deal with his own feelings, he can't recover from the emotional dimension of his cardiac crisis. The greater your fear, the more the patient pushes himself, ignoring prescribed physical limitations. The more you express concern about heart-healthy diet, the more stubborn he gets, refusing to give up fatty foods.

Caring about your mate doesn't mean doing everything for him at the expense of your own needs. And genuine caring involves letting go and encouraging your mate's independence.

Ultimately, it is not your responsibility to make your spouse recover. You can help. You can be supportive. And you can care. *But you do not have the power to save his life.* No person can take that basic responsibility for another.

Here is a Heartmates® checklist to help you discern between caring and caretaking:

Caring	Caretaking
Spontaneous	Calculated
Free	Controlling
Confident	Stems from helplessness
Motivated by love	Motivated by insecurity
Unlimited	Conditional

Responsibility and the Male Cardiac Spouse:
A Note to Husbands

Heart disease is the number one killer of men in the United States. But men rarely worry about their wives having heart attacks. According to the most current statistics, only one in six heart attack victims are women. But in the past fifteen years we have seen a dramatic rise in the statistics of female cardiac patients. This may be due in part to the rising number of women who smoke, as well as to the increasing number of "type A" women who participate in stressful careers.

As a male cardiac spouse, you have special and unique needs. Besides being part of a minority, coping with your wife's illness presents difficult challenges. You share some common concerns with female cardiac spouses, most specifically, the deeply held hope that your mate will recover. But when it comes to dealing with the day-to-day details of recovery, your paths diverge.

There are a number of special issues that set you apart. On an emotional level, it may be difficult for you to express your feelings. Just as women in our culture have been taught to suppress their needs, men have been taught to cover up their feelings. Consequently, your first response to seeing your wife in danger and in pain is to present a "strong" front. While some men feel comfortable expressing feelings, most are inhibited or embarrassed about appearing frightened or sad. On the inside you may feel devastated; on the outside you remain stoic. Maintaining a "macho" image increases your stress. What you really need is to let down your guard and allow yourself to feel your pain.

By and large, men have been educated to be breadwinners. In our culture it is rare for a man to take on the role of caretaker. Men learn early, from their mothers, to expect caretaking from women. Tradition dictates that men are providers; women are nurturers.

In a cardiac crisis, the roles are reversed. From the moment your wife is diagnosed as having heart disease, you find yourself in the position of caring for her. Without training or preparation, you are expected to have an instant aptitude for nursing, household maintenance, even childcare.

If you feel frightened and overwhelmed by suddenly becoming the primary caregiver, you're not alone. Most male cardiac spouses feel overwhelmed by the new demands thrust upon them. It's not a question of whether you care, but of *how* to express your concern. In some ways, it's a matter of style. It's not unusual to hear a male cardiac spouse say that just sitting at the hospital is difficult and that he'd rather express his caring in a more active way. Even the most devoted husband may feel pressured by his wife's need for emotional support.

On a practical level, being a male cardiac spouse can seem like suddenly arriving in a foreign country. This may become evident on your first serious trip to the supermarket. Even if the layout of the store is familiar, having to find items low in sodium and cholesterol requires familiarity with a foreign language. If you survive the supermarket, the next stop is the kitchen, where the utensils are arranged according to some indecipherable code. Finding the tools and making a meal for a heart patient is stressful for all cardiac spouses. It's especially challenging for men who haven't had much experience cooking.

Dick, known to his family and friends as the strong, silent type, described how he struggled to express his caring and love to his wife. He had never been effusive, and, like many men of his generation, he was uncomfortable articulating his feelings. Dick loved Jean dearly. After her heart attack, he showed his concern by taking over all the household chores on top of his regular long hours at work.

He was particularly proud of how good he was at vacuuming. Three weeks into Jean's recovery, she resumed her housework, including vacuuming. She didn't appear to appreciate Dick's efforts or to realize that this was his way of expressing his love. Dick felt frustrated with Jean's perfectionism and frightened that she was pushing herself too much. Mostly he felt defeated.

Like all cardiac spouses Dick needed support and understanding. Asking for support is something else that may prove to be more difficult for men. It's natural for men to be shy, ashamed, or unwilling to ask for help, believing that it implies weakness. If you are holding back but need to ask for help—whether it's a hand with the cooking, or crying on someone else's shoulder—go ahead and ask. You're in an extremely vulnerable position right now. *You need and deserve all the support you can get!*

Flexibility is needed to deal with the new demands of being a male cardiac spouse. The pressures of trying to combine your career, housework, parenting, and caring for your mate, require perspective and an ability to shift gears. Your job may well be the source of the most pressure. If you're the primary or the sole breadwinner, you may feel tense about taking time off from work, especially with increased medical bills, and if your wife is not working during recovery.

The toughest thing may be realizing and accepting that *you can't do everything.* You need to reach out to family and friends and ask for help. It's only a myth that men have to handle everything alone.

From Patient to Partner

There are negative consequences of acting in an overresponsible way. Getting stuck in the rigid role of caretaker fosters dependency, which, in turn, may slow the physical recovery of your mate.

Many years ago the treatment for a heart attack was weeks, sometimes months, of bed rest. The most up-to-date information suggests that lying in bed weakens rather than strengthens patients. Muscles that aren't used tend to atrophy. Today, cardiac patients are encouraged to begin walking two or three days after a heart attack or after surgery.

Cardiac rehabilitation programs are based on a carefully modulated regimen of activity interspersed with rest. Trying to limit your spouse's physical activity by doing everything for him directly opposes modern medical wisdom.

When you take too much responsibility for your mate you hamper your own recovery. If you're continually taking care of him, you are probably not taking good enough care of yourself. And encouraging your mate's dependence can be psychologically and emotionally damaging.

Finally, attitude has a tremendous impact on recovery. Cardiac patients struggle with the challenge of holding on to their self-respect. Perception of self-worth can be negatively affected by the stigma associated with heart disease. Rebuilding a healthy self-image happens gradually, as your mate successfully handles more and more, and integrates realistic limitations.

A positive attitude takes motivation and confidence. If you persist in taking over for your mate, he may start to wonder if his condition is more serious than he's been told. Doing things for him that he's capable of doing for himself makes him feel handicapped and inadequate. After a while, an individual who sees himself as an invalid will begin to believe that he is truly "in-valid." No cardiac spouse wants to contribute to such a negative attitude.

Trapped in a situation of overresponsibility and caretaking is no way to meet either of your recovery needs. Both of you may be strained in a relationship that needs caring, not caretaking, and right responsibility, not overresponsibility. Stress levels in the relationship may have escalated. Both of you may feel smothered; neither feels supported.

If you feel that you're doing well sharing and balancing responsibilities—congratulate yourself! If not, the following five steps can help you start shifting responsibilities in a way that will enhance and strengthen your relationship.

HEARTMATES® FIVE STEP PLAN FOR RIGHT RESPONSIBILITY

Step 1: Accept your powerlessness. This is easier said than done, but it is the critical first step. Until you can accept that caretaking and controlling are running your life, you will be shortsighted and your perceptions will be distorted. Continuous attempts at managing the unmanageable will lead you to a dead end.

Step 2: Assess your situation realistically. You know more about your situation than any expert or outsider. Be realistic about what responsibilities are urgent, and which ones can be put aside. Don't downplay or overdramatize the seriousness of your situation.

Step 3: Look honestly at your own behavior. Without blame or self-deprecation, analyze what you are doing and evaluate the positive and negative consequences to you, to your mate, and to your marriage.

Step 4: Differentiate between right and overresponsibility, caring and caretaking. You may want to discuss steps three and four with your spouse or a confidante you trust, to help you determine these differences.

Step 5: Make changes. The direction of change should be relative to where you are in recovery. As time passes, and you move farther away from the acute period of physical care, you need to begin to shift your attention from your mate's health to your own. Your recovery reestablishes your sense of self-worth and well-being, and opens you to real intimacy.

Wean yourself from the responsibility of being available for any and every demand. As the weeks and months go by, it is necessary to return to other aspects of life. At first the change may be small: leaving the house for a short time to do some shopping or take clothes to the cleaners. The next separate excursion may be lunch out with a friend, a concert, or community meeting. It may be advisable to build up to a bigger separation, like taking a retreat weekend, or visiting one of your grown children for a few days.

These steps are part of your recovery process. They take time, effort, commitment, and courage. No change comes easily. Lifelong habits conditioned by early training and cultural acceptance are very difficult to change.

Don't underestimate the healing power of sharing these issues with others who are in similar straits. Find someone you trust to cheer you on. Celebrate as you take steps to further your personal recovery.

Heart Disease Is a Family Affair

A family is an extension of marriage. Connected for better and for worse, in sickness and in health. When one member of a family is wounded, each individual is indelibly scarred. Life with heart disease is truly a family affair.

A cardiac crisis deeply affects all members of your family. It is extremely traumatic for a child of any age to experience a parent's near-death. If your mate's parents are alive, they have suffered agonizing worry and pain over *their* child. Brothers, sisters, nieces, and nephews have all shared in the concern.

The cardiac crisis is also a wonderful opportunity. Inherent within it is the potential for increased intimacy, nourishment, and support in families. Everyone is more vulnerable and sensitive. At such times, family members may drop defenses, forgive old hurts, and reach toward each other with caring and love.

123

Waiting during bypass surgery was excruciating. Our thirteen-year-old daughter, Debbie, chose to be at the hospital with me rather than go to school. We sat together surrounded by several dear friends.

By midmorning I felt restless and asked Debbie to go for a walk with me. Holding hands, we made our way to an island with one tree in the urban hospital block and stood together under the sun. I suggested that we do a visualization exercise for Marsh. We imagined the warmth and radiance of the sun entering the operating room, strengthening the surgical team, and filling the whole room with healing light. We visualized energy and prayers coming from our friends all over the country. We saw ourselves as a channel for energy flowing through us and into the hospital to Marsh and to the team repairing his heart.

I felt especially blessed to have a child who would share such a prayer with me. Later we decided we needed another walk, so we returned to our island. With traffic whizzing by, we closed our eyes and held hands again. This time Debbie led our personal meditation.

When the chaplain brought the news that the repair had been successful and "they were closing," Debbie and I held each other, our tears of joy and thankfulness mingling. Suddenly we were starving, and we celebrated with lunch.

It is ideal when family members can support each other in a crisis. Unfortunately this doesn't always happen. A crisis can also intensify conflicts and magnify misunderstandings. The family has the basic strength and resilience of any institution that maintains itself over generations. But within all families there are painful scars and unhealed wounds. A family crisis can offer an opportunity to heal old rifts and resentments.

The cardiac crisis automatically makes you the anchor of the family. It is your task to keep relatives informed. You are solely responsible for your children: their activities, school, appointments, meals, and other arrangements. It falls on you to respond to everyone's emotional needs.

The stress of being the family anchor may not at first be obvious. But consider the weight you're carrying on your shoulders. If you're like most cardiac spouses, you're preoccupied with your mate's recovery, and you're worried about how upset your children are. You may be concerned about where the next paycheck will come from, and the last thing you want is for your children to know you're worried. You're distressed about leaving your mate's side, and simultaneously feel burdened about not giving your children enough time and attention.

Anchoring your family makes you aware that all family members are affected by the cardiac crisis. It does *not* mean that you can fix every problem or that you're responsible for healing unpleasant or painful relationships among family members. Responsible leadership means appreciating the opportunity for renewed family unity. And leadership means accepting and respecting family members' needs as they too progress through the cardiac crisis.

Your children's emotional needs add to your stress and exhaustion. You have to inform your child of the family crisis. Adult children should be informed as soon as possible. But even this general rule has its exceptions.

Dana feared that her daughter, Michelle, would have a miscarriage upon learning that her dad had experienced a heart attack. Michelle lived hundreds of miles away and was in the eighth month of a difficult pregnancy. Dana weighed the possible consequences of informing Michelle or withholding the information. She tried to take all perspectives into consideration: Michelle's need to see her father, his need to be comforted by his daughter, and the new baby's safe arrival.

Little or no attention is paid to the needs of the children of cardiac patients by school or other institutions that do provide help in cases of "defined" stress like divorce or the death of a parent. Unless your children openly express it, you may not be aware of what they are going through. My clients are routinely surprised when their children let them know how much the cardiac crisis has affected them.

"Cardiackids" are expected to be fine because their parent is recovering. In most cases, we either ignore or sweep aside children's feelings and concerns, either out of ignorance or because our own concerns are so consuming.

The cardiac crisis deeply affects children. Cardiackids have feelings they need to understand and express. They experience the fear of nearly being left without a parent, the guilt of believing they caused the cardiac event, and the shock of their secure world becoming permanently uncertain. Cardiackids need to talk out the powerful impressions and images that haunt their dreams and waking hours.

Changing Family Rules and Roles

Your position as a family anchor reaches beyond your children to members of your extended family. Relatives with whom you normally have minimal contact may be more visible than usual. Depending on how your family gets along, handling the relatives can be a blessing or a burden.

As the cardiac spouse, you are the liaison for all other family members. And regardless of your relationship with individual family members, each has genuine feelings toward your mate and a real stake in his recovery. You need to protect yourself and your mate and still respect other family members' needs.

Virginia, a forty-one-year-old cardiac spouse, had difficulty keeping Lyle's family's visits to a minimum. She was worried that he wouldn't tell his three sisters and their husbands and children when he was too exhausted to visit. Even though Virginia was the youngest in the family, she was efficient and tough. She established two periods during the day when guests could come. When visiting hours were up, she personally ushered everyone out.

One morning, after being told that Lyle was napping and couldn't be disturbed, his oldest sister asked to see Virginia's "cop's badge." The sister informed her, in no uncertain terms, that the family didn't appreciate being told when and for how long they could visit their own brother.

After the first three weeks, Virginia loosened the rules. She was surprised when Lyle asked her to reinstate the regime, saying he was glad she had protected him. He still tired easily and found it uncomfortable to ask guests to leave.

Making decisions that take everyone's needs into account is practically impossible. You must try to be sensitive to your mate's relatives, but at times your priorities are bound to clash.

Barbara, a devoted wife, complained that her mother-in-law was sabotaging the heart-healthy diet she had instituted since Arnold's bypass surgery. Twice a week, *every* week, Sarah continued to deliver the home-cooked treats that she had always made to please her son. Butter-laden pastries and salty soups were Sarah's specialties. And her cooking was delicious! Barbara understood that it was one way in which Sarah could express her love for her son. But she finally put her foot down: "Either heart-healthy recipes or no recipes." The new dietary rules included Sarah, and there would be no exceptions.

In a family crisis, it sometimes seems as if there are too many cooks in the kitchen. Usually passive relatives suddenly become opinionated when their loved one's health is at stake. Decision making gets complicated when affected family members differ as to appropriate action. As the cardiac spouse, the buck stops with you. You make the decisions. This demands all your assertiveness and a willingness to carefully weigh differing opinions.

Jon, a rather shy individual, described his dilemma after his wife, Lois, had a heart attack. Her family, large and vociferous, met every evening to hash over the pros and cons of Lois' treatment. When the cardiologist advised bypass surgery, Lois' family convened in earnest. Jon felt left out and impotent as they argued back and forth late into the night. They finally agreed on the "right" course of action, informing Jon that he should tell the doctor of their decision. At no point was his opinion solicited.

If you honestly believe that other family members are interfering with your mate's recovery, do whatever is needed to protect yourself and your spouse.

A word of caution: A family crisis can also be used to lay blame or to vent past bitterness. Monitoring of visiting hours or excluding close relatives from decision making—playing the "cop"—may disguise an unconscious desire to hurt.

Families act according to patterns that have existed and repeated themselves for generations. Each individual has unique roles in his or her family. When a family crisis hits, everyone automatically falls back on the old established roles. Sometimes these work well in helping the family cope. Or, old roles may snarl an already burdensome situation.

A thirty-two-year-old cardiackid explained how she and her sister fell into their typical roles after their mother's heart attack. One sister was in charge of cosmetic concerns; the other handled the emotional issues. The former went out and bought a new robe and nightgowns for their mother; she made sure her mom's makeup was fresh and her hair coifed to keep her spirits up. The latter translated the doctors' reports and facilitated communication among the three generations of the family.

All family members are needed during a crisis. Each member of your family is an individual with unique gifts. Appreciating each other's contributions is an essential part of pulling together. If one member of your family is best at interpreting medical information, he or she should handle that. If another has always been the clown, comic relief has its place too. All family members, simply by virtue of their love and concern, have a valuable and legitimate role in the process of recovery.

Major Issues Confronting Cardiac Families

The effects of the cardiac crisis on family members may not be readily apparent. On the surface, your family seems the same as usual. But it's *not* the same! The cardiac crisis forces change and reversal in family relationships, roles, and rules. The long, cold fingers of uncertainty touch every family member. With the loss of certainty comes the urge to control and the yearning for order in a world suddenly strange, frightening, and uncontrollable.

If you are a parent, you are no doubt worried about the effect of the cardiac crisis on your children. The basic human fear of being abandoned, of being left helpless and alone, is an immediate as well as long-range concern for cardiackids. Since the onset of heart disease may occur in young, middle-aged, or older people, the needs of children differ from family to family. Within your family, each of your children will have individual needs depending on age, personality, and role in the family.

Your children's reactions to the cardiac crisis may evidence themselves as exaggerations of their normal behavior, or as unusual behavior that is difficult to understand. Young children may act out their fears through play. You may notice your seven-year-old play doctor or ambulance driver, her way of making order of the chaos. Your ten-year-old may refuse to play with friends, suddenly becoming solicitous and parental, sensing your fatigue and vulnerability, reversing the normal role of parent and child. Your adolescent son, struggling to achieve manhood and fearful about losing his father, may take over and try to be "the man of the house." Your adult children, involved in the family business, may find decision making difficult when the authority figure is suddenly unavailable for counsel. Your independent, single daughter, usually too busy to talk, drops by every evening after work, disregarding her personal routine and social life.

Cardiac spouses will try to appear strong and competent so that their children will feel safe. You may assume a well-defended stance in order to get through the day. Ironically, when cardiackids see the facade of a strong, silent model, they get the message, "Don't ask! Don't talk about it." And they don't. This is especially true of adult children. Attuned to your stress level, they may try to cope with theirs by guarding their feelings closely. The only way children of all ages may know to be cooperative and helpful is by *not* demanding your attention, not rocking the boat.

Unaired feelings can fester and leave permanent scars. Once a cardiackid is shaken by the knowledge that his parent is mortal, he will never again be an innocent. The illusion of security is forever broken.

Edward, age fifty-eight, was twelve years old when his father suffered a heart attack. Whenever Edward and his brother made the least bit of noise, their mother would come out of the kitchen or bedroom, looking frightened, and say, "Shhh, shhh." Edward was terrified that his noise would kill his father. He became more and more withdrawn.

Recalling those days, Edward remembered that his family never talked about his father's illness or what was happening to them. One evening at the supper table his fear erupted. His question echoed through the kitchen. "Will Daddy die?" His mother pushed her chair away from the table and ran crying into the bathroom. The rest of the family finished supper in silence.

After more than fifty years, Edward's memories are still vivid. The trauma of having been a cardiackid returned when his wife Florence had a heart attack. Once he shared his memories and feelings, he was able to cope with the present.

Florence's heart attack was an opportunity for Edward to heal an old wound.

Role Reversals

Changes in family relationships occur as a result of the cardiac crisis. If the onset of heart disease means that the cardiac patient does not return to work, financial issues may affect the family dynamics. When adult children begin to help parents financially, it is the beginning of the role reversals that come with aging. Parents, used to being in charge, have to adjust to being progressively more dependent on their children.

Margaret, a cardiac spouse, was concerned about her eleven-year-old son. Ever since Rob's dad suffered a heart attack, Rob had assumed responsibility for all the physical work around the house. Snow-shoveling is a major undertaking in their northern winter.

On the surface such a change in family responsibility seems simple and uncomplicated. Each winter tensions arise in the family. Rob's dad feels guilty that he is physically unable to shovel and must leave the entire job to Rob. He paces from window to window, scrutinizing Rob, watching every flake he moves. When he's finished, Rob saunters in, proud of the job he's done, hoping he will hear praise from his dad. His father, unable to express his guilt, either criticizes the quality of Rob's work, or comments on how he ought to have done it. The scene usually ends with Rob slamming the door to his room and isolating himself for the rest of the day. And since each year brings new snow, winter continues to be a stormy time, symbolizing the changes that heart disease has brought their family.

Less dramatic but just as painful is the change of lifestyle as aging parents become more dependent on grown children who are busy with their own families and careers.

Sunday dinners and holiday celebrations, long the pride of the parents, move down to the next generation. Children may need to arrange for their parents' doctor visits, transport them when they can no longer drive, and take charge of their Sunday outings.

The stress of this transition is difficult for all family members. Children may take over tasks lovingly or grudgingly, and parents may give them up graciously or stubbornly. All of these changes can be difficult to face and accept. Professional counseling can help improve coping and communication skills.

Many cardiac couples find it a difficult adjustment to accept help, especially from their children. For most of us, receiving is harder than giving. You and your mate may find yourselves in the "sandwich generation," between your grown children and your aging parents. When your focus and energy are directed toward coping with the cardiac crisis, carrying the responsibility for aging parents adds more stress to an already overwhelming situation.

If you are sandwiched between aging parents and growing children, you need to decide where to put your energy. You may be accustomed to the role of caregiver, but with the additional energy required to deal with the cardiac crisis, you may be unable to give as much as usual to your children *or* your parents. The young and the aged may be unprepared or unable to give you the care you need right now.

Don't be reluctant to ask for help from other members of the extended family at this time. *You cannot do it all yourself!* And members of your family need to give, too. Even young children can make worthy contributions and find comfort in being needed. Other sources of help are available through your local social service agencies. Don't hesitate to ask for the assistance of the social worker at your hospital to connect you with the appropriate agency.

Dealing with Cardiackids

Your love for your children makes you naturally concerned about their reaction to the cardiac crisis. Perhaps you feel that you must be more in charge than usual in order to compensate for their feelings of insecurity. You are the one who will assume the role of intermediary between your children and your sick spouse, keeping each filled in on how the other is doing.

Juggling your needs for privacy and support with your children's increased demands is a tricky balancing act. You want to be there for them at a time when you are struggling to be there for yourself.

The impulse to protect your children from pain and anguish is universal. But the truth is, it's impossible to do so. The cardiac crisis has occurred. You, your mate, *and* your children have been and will continue to be affected. Even if you could protect your children from hurt, it wouldn't necessarily be doing them a favor. Learning how to cope in a crisis is a valuable part of growing up.

There is no such thing as a perfect parent. And the pressure of being a cardiac spouse makes parenting even more challenging. If you're not as patient and responsive as usual, keep in mind that you are parenting alone, without your main source of support, your mate.

My rule of thumb in dealing with children is to remember that *kids are people too*. In a cardiac crisis, children have questions, and they have feelings. A child of any age has the right to be informed about what is happening to his or her parent.

•   •   •

Your Children's Right to Know

Adult children don't have the same access to hospital staff that you do. They aren't around as much as you are, and doctors and nurses may not take their questions seriously. Hospital regulations might prohibit young children from visiting at all.

Nothing is more fearful than the unknown. Even though you may not understand the details of every conversation you have with the medical staff, you do experience some relief from being given regular progress reports and information. Your children may not understand every detail either, but they will feel included and reassured if they are also informed.

Sometimes children get the idea that they are superfluous or in the way during the cardiac crisis. If you keep them apprised of discharge plans and recovery programs, they will feel more free to ask other questions they might have.

You must be the liaison between your children and your spouse. At times this arrangement may offer the only option. But nothing is as satisfying as direct contact between them. As soon as your mate is moved from cardiac care to a recovery unit in the hospital, you can arrange daily phone communications between him and his young children. Calls need not be long, but it is affirming and encouraging to hear Daddy's voice. Sharing a good-night kiss over the phone is better for both than none at all.

Over the long term, it is important for you to step away from negotiating family relationships. Trying to improve other's relationships doesn't work. You may be tempted to step in and help when you see your spouse and your adult children striving to establish communication. They may have conflicts to resolve, new things to talk about, or love to express to each other. Give them the space to do so without interference.

Questions from your children for which you have only tentative answers or none at all can distress you. Inviting your children's questions does not mean that you know the answers. Feel free to respond with three simple words, "I don't know."

The most feared question of course is, "Is my Daddy going to die?" The truth is that you don't know for sure. You might want to cloak the issue and respond only with the data and statistics that you have heard at the hospital. But a real question needs an answer from your heart as well as your mind. Your response might be, "Chances are, since Daddy has lived through the first forty-eight hours after a heart attack, that he will recover. I sure hope so, although I don't know for sure, and even the doctors can't be certain. I know that you're really scared and I feel afraid too." Such an answer may be followed by a long hug, shared tears, a special prayer.

What if you are ready and willing to answer your children's questions, but they remain silent? The most effective way to respond is to be open and accessible. Forcing children to talk about their feelings will only make them more resistant. Each of your children will deal with the cardiac crisis in an individual way.

Our family had a week to plan before Marsh's bypass surgery. Debbie decided immediately that she wanted to be with me in the hospital. She said she would be unable to concentrate and would find it intolerable to be sitting in school while her Dad was being operated on.

Our fifteen-year-old son, Sid, reacted in an opposite way. He thought it would be unbearable to sit in the hospital for hours. His preference was to be at school and be distracted from the surgery.

Sid worked out an elaborate plan for being informed. His idea was to run home from school and hear the phone ringing as he unlocked the front door. We agreed on the exact minute that I would call, and we synchronized our watches. And that was how Sid received the news that his Dad had come through the surgery successfully.

I was surprised at how differently our two children reacted. I particularly appreciated that each of them knew exactly what they needed on that stressful day.

Your children may tell friends their account of what happened to them and their parent during the cardiac event. You know from your own experience that telling and retelling your story is a necessary review that helps you integrate and understand what happened. Your children's versions of the experience may be different than yours. Restrain, if you are able, the urge to "correct" them.

As they share their feelings, you may feel it's up to you to "make your kids feel better." You don't have the power to do that. You can only trust the storytelling process to help your children come to a sense of order and peace about such confusing and chaotic experiences.

Helping Your Children Heal

Children need to be encouraged to speak about the frightening images they have. Like telling a nightmare, it's important to bring the dark and frightening memory into the light. Such images may never be forgotten, but saying them aloud can help divest them of their power.

When given the opportunity, most cardiackids are eager to talk about their experiences and images. One young man said that he couldn't get free from the horrible image of his mom straining against the respirator. A teenager described her pain and shock seeing her father so vulnerable in the cardiac care unit after a heart attack. An adult cardiackid explained his paralysis in decision making in the family business because his image of his father was of the perfect businessman. He was sure that he would make an irreversible mistake. He confronted his feelings of inadequacy as he moved toward the inevitable, the younger generation taking over the work of the patriarch.

Rarely do cardiac families talk about how the cardiac patient looked after open heart surgery. The sounds of the respirator and the numerous monitoring devices; the sight of countless tubes coming in and going out of the patient's body, neck, and nose; the antiseptic smells and the chill of the patient's flesh are too much to assimilate. The technology may be sophisticated, and the techniques may be routine, but when a spouse and children of any age see their loved one in this state they may respond with horror, terror, or despair. If the unspoken rule is "say nothing" or "keep a stiff upper lip," each family member suffers alone.

A cardiac spouse expressed concern that for months her nine-year-old son, Bobby, cried every time he heard an ambulance siren. I suggested she ask him what the sound reminded him of, and that she respond to Bobby from her heart. Bobby told her that the sound reminded him of seeing his daddy being taken away in the dark night by a screaming ambulance. He didn't think he would ever see his dad again. Bobby sat on his mom's lap and they had a long hug. Then they talked about how scary that time had been for everyone in the family, and how lucky they all were that dad had recovered. Happily, after their talk, Bobby stopped crying at the sound of a siren.

Making yourself available to share your feelings with your children can be a relief for all of you. There is no need to hide your honest emotions. Express your feelings openly and encourage your children to do the same. Shared family tears soothe and heal.

Children in cardiac families may need an expanded foundation of support during the cardiac crisis. If you have children of school age, I recommend you tell your children's teachers about the cardiac crisis. Information that deepens a teacher's understanding of what occupies your child's thought is useful. Your child's teacher can be a symbol of stability during a time of emotional confusion and family change. An adult ally outside the family can be a teenager's supportive listener.

Informing teachers may include educating them about the cardiac crisis, telling them that it *is* a family crisis, even though cardiac recovery is expected. Remember, bypass surgery has come to be seen as a routine procedure—with over 500 bypass operations done everyday in the United States, it is the most common surgery done today. Recovery from heart attacks is thought to be occasion for celebration and gratitude. Let the teachers know that your children are experiencing a family crisis. Each family member is in the process of understanding and accepting a new reality; such change requires time and patience. Children have serious questions and experience feelings which need to be encouraged and supported by sensitive adults.

Carla visited her daughters' parochial school when Patrick needed bypass surgery. She wanted the teachers to be prepared in case the girls reacted unusually. Carla was pleasantly surprised to find that her eight-year-old, Marie, had already told her teacher. In fact, she had asked that a prayer for her dad be included in the regular morning prayer. Next, Carla visited her ten-year-old's teacher. The teacher knew nothing about the family crisis and was glad to be informed so she could be helpful. Carla returned home confident that the girls' teachers would do everything in their power to help.

Dealing with young, and grown, children over time requires a basic understanding of the nature of the cardiac crisis. Although your children are different from you, each a unique individual, they will go through a similar process as they cope with the cardiac crisis. Universally, family members experience disruption, shock, confusion, anxiety, fear, and anger, and eventually accept a new family life that includes heart disease. They may exhibit and express their reactions differently, but they too are recovering from a crisis.

It takes time for cardiackids to come to terms with heart disease in the family, but children naturally and gradually return to more normal behavior. In some cases, however, the cardiac event results in more serious, long-term problems.

What are danger signals that indicate your child is stuck in the crisis and needs help? Because each child is unique, it is not easy to define "normal" progress. Take into account how long particular behavior continues, and how your child's actions differ from before the cardiac crisis. Remember that you know your child better than anyone. If you sense that he or she is having serious problems, trust your judgment. Here are some warning signals:

Angry outbursts
Dramatic changes in their marks at school
Behavior problems at school
Persistent nightmares
Lethargy and/or exhaustion
Clinging to parents
Crippling fears
Withdrawal and/or isolation

If you believe your child is suffering from any one or a combination of these behavioral signals, don't hesitate to consult a school social worker or psychologist. Another resource is your local hospital's social service department. You may find that there are professionals or programs available to your child at school or at the hospital. Many high schools have groups for students who are experiencing unexpressed grief or family stress. Expert advice doesn't supplant your influence; it supplements it.

Here is a guide to help you evaluate your family members' needs as they deal with the cardiac crisis. It includes reminders and hints to improve communication within the family. You will also find suggestions for getting help and support for your family.

HEARTMATES® FAMILY NEEDS ASSESSMENT GUIDE

1. Does each family member *know* that it is normal far *all* family members to be affected by the heart disease of *one* of its members? If not, how can such an understanding come about?

• Get more information.
• Ask more questions.
• Have more discussion among family members.
• Express feelings.
• Share this guide, chapter, or book with family members.

2. How aware and supportive are you to each of your children's reactions to the cardiac crisis? You might want to think about the initial and long-range reactions of each family member. Remember, no response is better than any other. Here is the perfect moment to value and appreciate the individual qualities of each member of your family.

3. Do family members ask questions and comment on concerns that are important to them individually within the family? If not, how can this need be met? Here are some suggestions to help relax the code of silence that may exist within your family:

At your next family get-together (Sunday dinner, a visit, or a prearranged family meeting) ask directly if anyone has questions about your spouse's present condition, past cardiac events, or future plans.

Establish a question box in the kitchen that can be opened regularly at a time when all family members are present. Let questions be asked anonymously, if family members aren't able to ask aloud.

Be willing to share your questions too. You don't have to understand it all perfectly. Other family members may be able to offer new perspectives.

4. How do you inform your children about the difficulties you are having?

• Do you say how you feel?
• Do you ask them to listen to you?
• Do you solicit their opinions and advice as you confront necessary and difficult decisions?
• Do you allow your children to give to you (physically, emotionally, financially)?

5. Does each family member have someone outside the family to talk to regarding the cardiac crisis? Is the listener available often, regularly, or seldom? Is the listener an extended family member, a friend of approximately the same age, a special adult, a mentor, a spiritual guide?

6. Have you let others offer support to you and your family?

• Inform your children's teachers.
• Let your minister, rabbi, or priest know of your family crisis.
• Contact your hospital cardiac rehabilitation staff to get support for family issues.
• Seek help from a family therapist or social service agency specializing in family concerns.

Simply wanting your family to become more intimate isn't enough to make it happen. Family patterns are established over long periods of time, often passed down through generations. Consequently, change is slow—one step at a time. Even positive change includes the element of uncertainty, so it can be strange and, in some ways, rather frightening.

During the process of recovery, anything uncertain can feel threatening. Go slowly. And remember: You alone are not responsible for all the other members of your family. As much as you may want the cardiac crisis to be a catalyst for closeness, you can't make other people change. They have to be motivated, too. Concentrate on how you can be available to give and receive from members of your family.

Concerning Blended, Broken, and Alternative Families

Heart disease does not confine itself to the ideal American family, a loving couple with 2.4 children. It strikes blended families, separated and divorced couples, and couples who are not married. These family configurations convolute an already complex situation. Family therapists say that once there are children, there is no such thing as divorce. Events that impact upon families—and surely heart disease is one of these—mark all family members, past and present.

SEPARATION AND DIVORCE

As a former spouse of a cardiac patient, your concerns will run the gamut from responding emotionally to your ex-spouse's heart disease to wondering how to help your children. You probably have at least some of the following questions: Shall I visit at the hospital? Why do I feel sad, angry, or afraid when we're no longer married? Is it appropriate for me to share my feelings with the patient? With our children? How should I act in relation to his family?

How can I interact with his present spouse? What is the most supportive position I can take for our children in a family crisis from which I'm isolated, or about which I have unresolved feelings?

My advice in these matters is simple, but not neccssarily easy: Act from your heart! There are no right or wrong answers. Etiquette and protocol don't reach into this realm. If there is anything unresolved between you and your exspouse, there may be criticism no matter what you do.

Try not to judge or censor your feelings. You are entitled to respond any way that seems right. You may also decide to use the opportunity of the cardiac crisis to reconcile old differences. That is perfectly appropriate. Hard feelings may soften at a time when heart disease has made all of you more vulnerable. And then again, nothing may change between the two of you.

No matter how you feel toward your ex-spouse, try your best to respect your children's relationships with him. If your children's loyalty has been a point of contention, a family crisis can escalate it. Your children's love should not be something to fight over. Children should never have to shoulder the burden of your pain and anger with each other. They have a right to their own personal relationship with each of you.

If you feel unwelcome or too awkward to visit at the hospital or at home during recovery, call a member of your ex-spouse's family to arrange a visit for your children. It may be hard to accept that your children need something that you aren't in a position to give. But there's more to being a good parent than meeting their every need. If that is the case, arrange for them to connect with grandparents or aunts and uncles who can function as their confidantes or provide them the "warm fuzzies" such a difficult situation requires.

UNMARRIED HEARTMATES

If you are a heartmate outside the legal tie of marriage, your situation poses questions of a different sort. Family members who rally round your sick heartmate may not even know about you or that your relationship exists. If they do, they may not appreciate the nature of your relationship or realize that you are deeply affected by your heartmate's illness.

If your relationship is secretive, your contact may need to be clandestine or even temporarily cut off. The cardiac crisis may be an opportunity for the two of you to consider the emotional costs of keeping your relationship from your families. Since heart disease is incurable, and potentially life-threatening even when recovery is complete, you may consider a change in the terms of your relationship.

Also to be discussed are financial arrangements for your future. Financial planning may change due to the cardiac crisis. If your heartmate has been providing financial support, it may be impossible for this to continue. Going through a cardiac crisis may give rise to new values, affecting the way you deal with money in your relationship.

Your participation in giving your heartmate physical and emotional support during recovery is more difficult if you are unmarried. If your loved one is part of his own family, your visible involvement in his recovery probably won't be welcome. If you are openly involved with, but not living with, a cardiac patient, the logistics of maintaining two households make support more complicated.

As an extralegal cardiac spouse, you will be doing your grieving and adapting without the safety or foundation that a family normally provides. No matter the reason why you've not married, you suffer during the cardiac crisis like all heartmates do. Seek out people who can be supportive to you, and who will listen to your concerns. Professional counseling is of practical help when your needs require confidentiality.

Family Heartache

When a family gets stuck in the process of recovery—when communication is essentially shut off, so that issues are not being confronted—natural healing doesn't happen.

The scenario of a "stuck" family may resemble the following story: Several months of "recovery" have passed. Father, the cardiac patient, feels depressed and is irritable and demanding. Mother, the cardiac spouse, feels resentment and is fatigued and overworked. The eldest daughter, who temporarily dropped out of college when her father suffered his heart attack, has neither looked for a job nor made arrangements to continue her schooling. The second child, a sixteen-year-old high school junior, is coming home late at night. His sullen and silent style has become exaggerated, and his grades have fallen. The youngest child, an eleven-year-old girl, is afraid to go to bed without a light on, and is often heard crying or screaming with nightmares.

No one mentions what is happening to any one individual in the family. No one notices that the family as a unit is failing to support its members. The crisis seems to have fragmented the family system and the children are acting out the pain that the father and mother are neglecting to address.

Sometimes school will call attention to a symptom by reporting falling grades or by commenting on behavioral changes in a child. It is a mistake, however, to focus on a child, officially labeling a symptom of family dysfunction as an individual problem or illness. Instead, the cardiac couple should be encouraged to face the issues directly. If they can, the children will be liberated from the obligation of carrying the unexpressed anger and pain of their parents.

Short-term consultation with a family therapist is the most appropriate help for a cardiac family. The family therapy perspective will protect an individual family member from becoming the erroneous focus, obscuring the real family issues opened by the cardiac crisis. Brief intervention is frequently all a family needs to break through the code of silence.

When parents are able to relate how frightened they are about having heart disease or how grateful they are for recovery, it has magical effects on all family members. When everyone acknowledges fear, the chances are that their hearts will open to each other, and the family can become a secure place for everyone. In a safe environment, family members can ask their questions and can voice their feelings.

The cardiac crisis offers more than just an opportunity to test a family's power to withstand and ward off pain. When hearts are physically and emotionally wounded, as all hearts are in a cardiac family crisis, there is a chance for the basic strength of the family to grow and for love to expand.

Not all families need professional help. A technique that can help is visualization. Here is a Heartmates® exercise that you can do alone, or you can invite your family to participate. Have someone read the exercise aloud each time you do it to avoid interruption.

HEARTMATES® VISUALIZATION:
A HEALING FAMILY MEETING

Find a quiet and comfortable place to sit. Close your eyes. Let yourself breathe normally, and relax. Imagine that with each inhalation you breathe in energy and with each exhalation you let go of tension. Continue to focus on your breathing until you feel calm and alert.

Now imagine a room in your home that is the warmest and most comfortable for your family. It may be your kitchen, den, or porch. Notice its furnishings and what makes it warm. See it awaiting and welcoming your family. And now, in your mind's eye, see all your family seated in a circle in this comfortable room. Everyone seems to know why they're here. The atmosphere is hopeful and cooperative.

You begin your family meeting by everyone holding hands as you sit in a circle. Together you share a silent prayer of gratitude for recovery, and a petition for family cohesion and individual strength. As much as you can, experience the feeling of all of you together in this moment of silence. As you complete the prayer, everyone drops hands, and an atmosphere of respect and concern settles over the room. There is a sort of peace, an aura of acceptance and protection that falls over the family.

Now imagine that without blame or shame, each family member speaks in turn about one personal concern. You listen with your heart to what each family member says. You, in turn, hear your own contribution with your heart as well. There is no verbal response to any statement that is made, but there is respect in the listening and there is caring from each to all.

Imagine that as each person speaks, the weight of the family is lightened and the light in the room gets brighter. The air the family is breathing is fresh and clean. You can smell growing grass and blossoming flowers.

Now, as the meeting ends, you sense family members really seeing one another. Each member is respectful of other family members' rights and abilities to deal with the crisis in their own ways and by their own timetables. Some affection may be expressed.

Everyone agrees to meet again soon. Your favorite room empties. You experience realistic hope about your family's ability to cope with the cardiac crisis.

You again focus your attention on your own breath. Gradually return to your present reality. Continue to breathe fully and naturally. Return, renewed, to the present.

Recovery and Hope for the Cardiac Family

How can you see opportunity in the cardiac crisis? "In the light of our everyday world, we cannot see the stars."[1] So much of your energy goes into just coping with the minute-to-minute and day-to-day changes. Everything you wish is focused on the past: You wish this had never happened, that the family would return to normal. Recovery and healing is a natural part of the cardiac crisis, too.

The power of the cardiac crisis has jolted and shocked everyone. Each member of the family needs to recover, and the family as a whole needs to heal. What can you do? The essential elements of every recovery include communicating, expressing feelings, understanding the meaning of the crisis, and supporting one another through the grieving process. Build an environment that honors individual differences and permits each person his own responses. Make space for every family member to cooperate.

For each family, the cardiac crisis presents something different; and the timing of healing is its own. Your family will move at its own pace and in its own way toward recovery.

The cardiac crisis can be regarded as an opportunity for reconnection within the family. A crisis can strengthen family bonds. Being there for one another puts "heart" into the family. Your reward will be enhanced respect and deepened trust, the goal of cardiac family recovery.

A Note to Cardiackids

As a cardiackid, your special concerns are different from your parents'. Perhaps you have been fortunate in having someone outside the family to talk with about the changes that are taking place. Or maybe you feel confused and alone. As a counselor and the mother of two teenage cardiackids, I'd like to offer you the following guidance:

1. You have a right to know what is happening. Depending on your age and your role in the family, you may or may not have been given sufficient information about what is going on. You are entitled, no matter how old or young you are, to know your parent's condition and prognosis. The cardiac crisis is real; your life is affected. *Ask the questions you need answers to.* You may have to ask your parents because you don't have direct access to doctors and other professional personnel. If you can't get the answers from your parents, ask others in your family—older brothers and sisters, cousins, aunts and uncles. There is nothing more difficult than dealing with the unknown. Some things just can't be known or predicted, but you should get whatever information exists. It is okay to ask any question that you have, even if there isn't an answer available. Remember to ask your questions again later, or to go to someone else if you don't get a satisfactory answer right away.

2. Accept your feelings and find ways to release them. All the feelings that you experience are normal. Most cardiackids have different feelings at different points of the crisis. You may go back and forth between feeling sad and happy, afraid and anxious, angry and guilty. All of these feelings are okay.

If your family is one that is uncomfortable talking about feelings, find other constructive ways to express yourself. Keep a diary or a journal and regularly write about how you feel. Talk with your friends. Search for an adult who will listen to you. Perhaps your favorite teacher, coach, or an activity leader whom you respect will take the time to hear you out. At a time like this, your special relationship with a grandparent can be good for both of you.

It really is important for you to express your feelings. Keeping them locked up inside can freeze the natural development of your relationships with your family and other people, too.

3. Don't blame yourself. Cardiackids sometimes believe that their behavior caused their parent's illness. That is not true! If you blame yourself, you will act overly careful and withhold your feelings—and that won't help anyone. If somebody tells you that you can cause a fatal heart attack by making a lot of noise, or that angering the patient will do him harm, don't believe it. Your feelings and behavior cannot cause a heart attack.

4. Don't be ashamed. If you sense that your parent is "damaged" or no longer a whole person because of heart disease, you may feel ashamed of that parent, of your family, even of yourself. But having a disease, or having physical limitations, doesn't make a person less whole. All human beings have dignity, regardless of their physical form. (This is the truth illustrated in the films *The Elephant Man* and *Mask*.)

5. It takes a while to return to normal thinking and functioning after a crisis. The cardiac crisis will affect you in ways you might not expect. You may have problems paying attention in class long after your parent is home from the hospital. Plan for more time than usual to do your homework. If you find that you can't think clearly, don't push yourself. Stop studying and go for a bike ride, shoot some hoops, talk on the phone, or take a warm shower. When you go back to the books, be gentle with yourself. You may even want to get permission from your teachers to turn some assignments in late. I'm not suggesting that you use the cardiac crisis to procrastinate or to get special privileges. Taking good care of yourself may require you to ease some of the stresses that you would otherwise handle effectively under normal conditions.

6. Roles and responsibilities in the family are changed by the cardiac crisis. You may be aware of the typical role that you and your brothers and sisters play in your family. If you are the "good child" in the family, you may find yourself really "wiped out" from taking on extra tasks and jobs to help your parents. If you are the "shy one" in the family, you may find it hard to get the information you need and even harder to talk about how you feel. Most people fall back on their typical roles to get through a crisis. It is not the best time to experiment with a new way of interacting with your family, but go for it if you can. A crisis is a time when everything is anything but familiar, so it is possible to try new modes of relating.

You also are likely to notice that your parents' roles have switched, maybe temporarily and maybe permanently. Your dad may have taken over the kitchen since your mother's surgery. Or Mom may have become more of a disciplinarian since Dad was hospitalized. Your parents may be struggling with new and different responsibilities and may seek your help. You may have to get up early before school to shovel the driveway, or take over the jobs your dad usually does, like changing screens and storms on the windows of your house.

New responsibilities, even temporary ones, can make you feel terrific. It is natural to care when your family is in crisis, and you can show some of that by being responsible and helpful. Putting a younger brother to bed, cleaning up the kitchen, or mowing the lawn is just exactly what you need to do to show your parents you care. Such tasks are practical and measurable and can give you the reassuring sense that the family can count on you when so much seems strange and confusing. On the other hand, you may resent having to take on extra responsibility, especially if you don't have any say in the matter, but it will give you a way to help your changing family.

In an ideal family all of these changes would be discussed and accepted before they happened. But no family is ideal, and it is more likely that you are assigned, sometimes without words, responsibilities that may burden you.

7. Try to understand your parents. Conflict between your parents may have escalated since the cardiac crisis. Their differences and different reactions to the crisis increase the tension between them. Whether they tell you so or not, it is important for you to know that they also feel helpless, out of control, frightened, sad, and angry about the cardiac crisis.

8. It is not your responsibility to take care of your parents. Even though you may want to alleviate the tension that you feel within the family, *you can only change yourself. You can't change other people.*

If your parents are separated or divorced, you may feel caught in a loyalty bind. You may live with your mother and depend on her to take you to see your father. It is an awkward situation, but one in which you owe it to yourself to do what your heart tells you. Staying close to your cardiac parent is your right, even if you don't live together. Discuss the situation with both your parents, letting them know that you love them both.

The deeper questions you must wrestle with concern your loss of innocence. You have seen that your parent is mortal, and now, the one thing you thought was secure, isn't. If your parent can die, then nothing in life is for sure. Remember when you realized there was no Santa Claus or Tooth Fairy? Your disappointment and sadness was real then—and now, too. You need time and space to mourn the loss of what you believed. Once you do that, you will have the opportunity to develop a more realistic foundation on which to build new trust. And that may lead you to appreciate just how precious your family and life itself are.

Sid, our son, was a senior in high school when he wrote the following essay. His assignment was to write about an event that had influenced his life. Sid rarely communicated his feelings verbally with the family. I had no idea that his father's heart disease had caused so profound a change in him. But his essay proved to me that images and memories need to be expressed if we are to overcome their hold on us. A cardiackid needs to express his feelings his own way, and in his own time. I was awed and moved as I witnessed Marsh's and Sid's hugs and tears after Sid read his essay to us one evening in our kitchen.

HE AIN'T HERCULES, HE'S MY FATHER

A soft placid sheet of snowflakes filled the skies on the cold winter evening. The scream of the ambulance snapped the peaceful hush of the night, but quickly became muffled. The screams remained in my mind long after. The ambulance held my father in its hollows while he fought for his life with a heart attack. Only minutes before, we were all sitting together watching "Monday Night Football." Now, my mother, sister, and I were watching the ambulance disappear into the night. Although I had always loved him, I never realized how valuable my father was to me until I almost lost him.

At age fourteen, I "loved" my father because he was my Dad; it was no more than the normal feeling a son has for his father. Nevertheless, he was my hero, and I looked up to him as a boy does to his favorite sports star. In high school, my father captained three sports: football, basketball, and baseball. He was the "All-city" quarterback and was voted the best athlete by his class. Through his mid-forties, he remained physically active, participating in softball, racquetball, and golf. He not only instructed me in the fine points of baseball, he also taught me how to wrestle by pinning me weekly during our "roughhousing matches." From my perspective, he was as close to Hercules as a man could get. I never had a foreshadowing of the disastrous event.

The hospital room was only steps away. I slowed my pace, afraid to see my wounded father. I peeked in and saw him: lifeless, with tubes going in and out of his body. His eyes opened when I entered the room, and when he made an effort to smile, I broke into tears. I could not believe that my hero was crippled. He was too weak to lift his hand to hold mine, so I grasped his hand and I held him, all of him, for the first time in my life. At that point, I realized how much I loved him! He was a supernova, an exploded star that had become thousands of times stronger and brighter.

After his hospitalization, my father returned home and didn't leave the house for another month. With my hero gone, a new relationship with my father dawned. His body had failed him; as time passed, he started to adjust. I learned what true disappointment was by watching the pain that he went through; it hurt inside to see him short of breath after climbing a flight of stairs.

Because of the threat that any day he could be gone forever, I have learned to value his presence whenever I am with him. I no longer take his "being there" for granted. No more do I worship my father as a hero. Rather, I observe with new eyes and have a greater understanding of who he really is. I watch him make mistakes, and I note his shortcomings. We discuss our daily lives, share humor, and compare our beliefs. My hero is gone. But I have a deeper feeling of love for the man that took his place.

Does Time Heal All Wounds?

My sense of my own identity was permanently changed when I became a cardiac spouse. I stopped believing that I had complete control over my life and my destiny. Marsh has heart disease. There is nothing I can do to alter that fact. I live in a world of imperfection, where change beyond my control occurs instantaneously.

I lost my innocence. Before Marsh's heart attack, I lived life as if it were an exciting adventure. I believed there were no limits to what Marsh and I could accomplish together. In one shocking moment, my naiveté was gone. Eventually a new reality was born in its place. I am neither invincible nor limitless. I am human.

I let go of my subconscious belief in immortality. Marsh's brush with death made me realize that our time on earth is limited, that we will not live forever. I had been squandering time as if I had eternity in my back pocket. I experience time differently now, treasuring each day, and I have learned to set my priorities more thoughtfully.

I gave up my trust that Marsh would always be there for me when I needed him. I had depended on his strength, his clarity, his wit, and his companionship for a quarter of a century. I had been oblivious to the impermanence of our relationship. I try now to appreciate what he gives me and not take his presence for granted.

My beliefs and dreams were gone. My wounds were so

*deep, I hurt to my very core. My pain has diminished with
time. Still, I'm sometimes reminded of it all when I look in the
mirror and see the lines in my face or the sadness in my eyes.*

Coping with heart disease is a pervasive, enduring,
and lifelong process. The original trauma may be past, but
there are permanent changes. Your body, mind, and spirit
have been scarred.

Fortunately, time is on your side. Your mate has
survived and so have you. As the weeks and months pass,
you are reassured more and more that life goes on. Time
has taught you a number of things. You're no longer afraid
to leave your mate at home, and you are less involved with
his physical symptoms. You've come through the crisis
with increased strength, resiliency, and adaptability.

But your journey isn't over. Everything has changed,
and even time can't make things "normal" again. You cannot erase what has happened. Our cultural conditioning
perpetuates the myth that if you just do everything right, all
will be fine; your pain will vanish and you'll live happily ever
after. But you're not living a fairy tale; this is your life. There
is no magic that can make the recent past disappear. There
are no pills or time machines to transport you back to an
earlier time of innocence. The cardiac spouse faces countless disappointments and broken dreams. Your spouse's
heart disease has affected your life-style, your financial
security, your marital relationship, and your most deeply
held beliefs.

You now question everything: your values, ideas,
and beliefs. If you have always believed that your husband
is stronger than you, his physical weakness and vulnerability caused by heart disease threaten this belief. If you've
measured your intimacy by the degree of passion in your
sexual relationship, new limitations may make you reevalu-
ate your perceptions. Firmly held ideas, like "Nothing bad
can happen if you believe in God," or "These things happen

to other people," are now meaningless, and you feel confused and betrayed. The cardiac crisis has upset your
security. Something is very, very wrong. You have reached
that universal and dramatic realization that *nothing will
ever be the same.*

Confrontation with permanent change can be devastating. Heart disease exacts its costs: limited activity, lost
security, and painful adjustments in your personal relationships. Your feelings of sadness and anger are valid, whether
they are in reaction to something small, like giving up your
favorite foods, or more profound, like relinquishing long-
term plans for the future.

Being a cardiac spouse forces you to remove your
rose-colored glasses. Your mate's heart disease has brought
you face to face with your own personal reality.

There is no cure for heart disease. What has happened is irreversible and permanent. Who can say why you
and your spouse have had to cope with heart disease? The
reasons are not always apparent; perhaps we must be faced
with challenges in order to change and grow. All change is
difficult, but not necessarily negative.

But just as there is no end without a beginning, there
is no loss without the hope of gain. In this case, there is a
positive path to traverse and a chance for personal growth.
The Tao's definition of crisis is "opportunity," and
Hippocrates said, "Healing is a matter of time, but it is
sometimes also a matter of opportunity."[1] *Carpe diem.*

Grief and Loss

Human life implies death and loss. Perhaps one of
the most difficult things we face is learning how to absorb
and survive loss—how to "let go."

Although grief is usually part of the emotional process following a death, it also can pertain to any change. To

accept the losses accompanying heart disease, you may need to grieve for your past, your life as it was before the cardiac crisis.

The custom of mourning is as old as life itself. And the past is rich with wisdom. The original Sanskrit definition of mourning means "remembering." In Greek, mourning means "caring." Mourning really includes both components. In order to work through your grief you must acknowledge and express the feelings generated by loss. You also need to "tell your story" and talk about your struggle in order to understand what has happened. Remembering and caring enable you to integrate and accept the loss.

Centuries ago, the rabbis of Judea codified rituals of mourning. The first year after a loss was divided into smaller parts: the first week, the first month, and the first eleven months. Observances and rituals for each period were defined, giving the family permission to mourn and providing a guide for "working through" grief.

Elisabeth Kübler-Ross, whose monumental work lifted the cultural taboo of silence about loss and death, suggested stages through which mourners pass, progressing from shock, disbelief, denial, and numbness through anger and depression toward acceptance.[2] Her analysis legitimized the process of grieving for many. People don't necessarily experience the stages in order; some move back and forth from stage to stage. Others experience several stages simultaneously. Even mourners who have reached the stage of acceptance may at times continue to wrestle with fears and yearn for the past.

Although professional literature has established the validity and therapeutic value of grief, there is still social pressure to keep the mourning responses brief. We are a people journeying in the fast lane, intolerant of anything that takes longer than the speed of light. Despite pressure to "hurry up and get on with life," it's essential to allow yourself time and attention to mourn. You may be at your most vulnerable, and need to proceed through grief at your own pace, without a model, a guide, or unqualified support.

The cardiac spouse's losses are real and important, though invisible to others and unvoiced by you. If you don't allow yourself to grieve, you will get stuck in a psychological rut. Resisting the natural process may even result in physical consequences, illness. Research has shown that natural immunity is reduced when someone experiences sudden and intense change; grieving people are more susceptible to disease for up to two years after a crisis.

Once you acknowledge that the cardiac crisis has wounded you, you can begin to look at your losses in earnest. Remember that your purpose is to heal and adapt from what *was* to what *is*.

The Healing Process

Healing requires time, but our culture is impatient. If your wounds were obvious, involving a scar or crutches, friends and family would better understand your need to take the time to heal. But your wounds are invisible. Judging by your surface appearance, everyone assumes that you are doing just fine. And in some ways, you are. But you still may be struggling to accept the permanent changes brought on by heart disease. Even if it means going against the grain, you need to permit yourself time to heal.

Healing is highly individual. Each person has individual needs and timing. Treat yourself kindly. Don't pressure yourself to rush through this. Don't push yourself faster than you can go, and don't let others, uncomfortable or impatient with your pace, pressure you into activities or decisions for which you're not yet ready.

Time is central to the healing process. But it alone isn't enough. You must also be willing to cleanse your wounds, i.e., confront your losses, rage, and mourn in order to come to terms with the reality of your life now. Forgiveness makes it possible to accept your imperfection, your spouse's, and the uncontrollable events that have happened. And the final step in healing is to turn from the process of introspection to reconnect with the world around you and look forward with anticipation as your present becomes the future.

Whether you are recovering from the trauma of chronic illness or the finality of death, the process of grief and healing is essentially the same. There are five basic steps in healing:

1. Recognizing your wounds
2. Facing reality
3. Releasing your feelings
4. Updating your images
5. Forgiveness

Recognizing Your Wounds

It's natural to try to escape pain. One way is to ignore what's happened. In some respects, that's easy to do. If your mate has had a full physical recovery, he may look healthier than he has in years. Recovered bypass patients often have ruddy complexions and report that they "feel great." A regular exercise program has probably made your spouse physically fit and more active than he was before his heart attack.

Some cardiac spouses try to avoid pain by trivializing it. You may tell yourself "this is no big deal" and attempt to live your life exactly as before. Other cardiac spouses are afraid of self-pity, continually asking, "What in the world have I got to complain about?" and denying themselves permission to examine very real wounds.

Don't try to escape pain—that only sends it underground. Wounds need fresh air to heal. Like an infection, pain continues to run its course, and cannot be cured with a band-aid or the casual pretense that it doesn't exist.

Don't deny reality—it won't help you heal. Denial hinders the recovery process and diminishes your freedom and spontaneity. An extreme but not unusual example involves Marilyn, the fifty-one-year-old wife of a cardiac bypass patient. Marilyn proudly described how she avoided her own painful feelings regarding Robert's surgery. She worked out a plan so that she would never see his scars. The last thing she wanted was to be reminded of the nightmare they'd been through. She made sure to be out of the bedroom when he was dressing or undressing. She got into bed only after Robert had turned out the light, so she wouldn't see his bare chest. If Robert went to sit by their apartment house pool in his swimming trunks, Marilyn would find something to do that kept her inside. This behavior required a great deal of energy and attention. What began as a solution ended up being a trap. Instead of diminishing her pain, Marilyn found that her life was dictated by her denial.

Recognizing your wounds may be difficult for several reasons, starting with the fact that you weren't raised to identify and value your own needs. You may be so conditioned to the role of caretaker that you honestly don't know that *you* have been hurt. A successful caretaker puts in twenty-four-hour days and every effort to take care of others and combat the inevitable. The caretaker doesn't know how to assess her own needs. She has been given no permission to let down or let go; the way she feels is the least of her worries. She's always on duty, perennially cheerful, and indefatigable, even after years of service.

But what will happen when you move beyond denial and habit to confront that deep and universal fear of the unknown? Will you survive if you remove the band-aids and see your wounds? Will you drown in your tears, or will they be a relief and a comfort? What proof is there that, if you look at what is lost, outdated, or gone, you will rise out of despair and chaos to something secure and meaningful?

Fear of the unknown can be fought only with faith and courage. You will never achieve peace of mind unless you come to terms with reality.

Courage is the price that life exacts for granting peace. The souls that know it not, know no release from little things.[3]

Recognizing your wounds does not guarantee positive growth. But if you have the faith that there is something beyond your pain, and the courage to act in the face of your fear, you will be closer to an acceptance of your reality.

Your pain is symptomatic of the losses you've experienced. *There is no way around pain; you must go through it.* Pain's partner, vulnerability, opens the door so you can look at yourself and your life. If you use all your energy to keep the door tightly shut, you will not heal. Your wounds will continue to fester and ooze, and your life will become more and more constricted with each passing month. You may never again have such an opportunity to evaluate your life, to take charge of what you want and need, and focus your energy to achieve new, more realistic goals.

Facing Reality

The second step in the process of healing is discerning what your loss means to you. A wound can heal only after its severity is determined. You must think about what has happened before you can figure out how you can heal.

One of the best ways to understand something is to talk about it. Seek out friends who will listen to you. Plan outings, like lunch in the back booth at your favorite restaurant or a secluded walk by the lake or in the woods, where you can talk undisturbed.

To fully grasp what you have lost, *review* (re-view) and *relive* your experience—it's an integral part of grieving. Begin at the beginning; tell a friend what happened to you. Each time you relate it, your story will change. As you try to understand, you may find that you need to get straight facts and information you have lost. Feel free to contact the doctor, family members, or anyone who might have the information you've missed or forgotten. Reviewing your experience helps you separate the reality of what has happened from your feelings about what happened. Keep talking. Over a period of time it will become clear to you how your life has changed.

As you talk, you'll begin to explore important questions that help you test what is real: "How does my spouse's heart condition really affect me? What is most important now in my life? What's realistic for me to expect of myself now? How do I feel about the ways in which our relationship has changed?" You need to lay a foundation for constructing a new, more realistic image of yourself. It helps, when you are testing what is real, to share your thoughts and ideas with a trusted friend who can give you another view, or respond in ways that deepen or broaden your perspective.

Releasing Feelings

Facing reality uncovers your feelings. At this point in the process, you begin to feel the anger, pain, and sadness associated with your losses. You may feel overwhelmed or out of control. But the pain of knowing is also cleansing. If you've been unable to cry since all this began, your tears may come now. Imagine them washing and cleansing your wounds; they offer relief, a loving gift to yourself. If you can, allow yourself to cry with someone you trust, who can give you support.

The release of emotion, through words and tears, helps heal your wounds. This may be an appropriate time to seek professional help. A skilled therapist can give you support, help you test reality, and listen to you.

Another release is writing. Keep a journal and use it to communicate with yourself. Set aside time everyday to sit in a comfortable place, tune into your thoughts and feelings, and write in your journal.

Remember, everyone who experiences loss, grieves. Your feelings indicate how deeply affected you are by your losses. Be aware of and accept your need to grieve; honor yourself and your life.

Many people believe that the outward expression of feelings is a sign of weakness. I contend that the opposite is true. It requires the utmost courage to express your feelings, and only the strong dare to do so. Shakespeare's advice in *Macbeth* applies to cardiac spouses today: "Give sorrow words; the grief that does not speak / Whispers the o'er fraught heart and bids it break."[4]

Anger is among the strongest of your feelings. Facing and paying attention to anger may feel to you like the first fatal step toward total disintegration. You wrongly tell yourself you can't risk that, because you have to stay strong to take care of your spouse and family.

Some cardiac spouses don't feel entitled to their anger. You weren't widowed by heart disease, so you have no right to be angry, you think. You may feel ashamed just touching on anger. One cardiac spouse told me that anger was a sin. When you feel wrong for being angry, admitting it can trigger a sense of unworthiness and low self-esteem.

Why bother with anger when it's so difficult? Why not sidestep it, accept and forgive? Because it's not possible! Anger is a normal human response to hurt and loss.

You can't reach acceptance without first dealing with your anger.

In order to let go of your anger, you must stop holding on to it, protecting it, and hiding it from yourself and others. Your anger may take the form of blame; you might blame the doctor, the professional staff, even the hospital system for how you feel or what's happened to you or your spouse. Your anger might be directed against your spouse for having heart disease, for smoking, for being a "type A, " or even for his inherited genetic factors. Maybe you're letting your anger smolder, resenting how your mate has treated you. Maybe you feel angry and hurt that your mate has withdrawn since all of this began. Maybe you feel emotionally deprived, sorely in need of care and affection. Or maybe you are furious that your spouse has not appreciated your extra effort on his behalf over these months.

If you were to express your feelings to your spouse, you might be amazed at how your perceptions differ. Even if you disagree, you still have to accept your anger. Your anger is based on *your* perception of your experience. You don't need to be fair, accurate, or unselfish. Holding on to your anger because you don't think it is "justified" will isolate you and put more distance between you and your mate. Sheltered anger also builds walls, shutting out friends' understanding and support.

Wives who relied on their faith before the cardiac crisis may find themselves angry at God. Helen, who had been very religious, felt as though God had turned His back on her. Another cardiac spouse, Caroline, described how unfair it was for God to abandon her after she had "been good" all her life. Yet another spouse believed that God was punishing her with the cardiac crisis.

People who live their faith, trusting their relationship with God, can afford to express their anger in words and tears. They don't need to keep their anger hidden inside. People abandon God by withholding their anger; by expressing it, they discover that God has been there for them all along.

Release of feelings doesn't happen in a day or a week; the process occurs over time and in small measures. You may hesitate to release feelings, certain that doing so will be overpowering. However, that is rarely the case. Your psyche, naturally healing itself, will determine a safe pace and protect the rest of your system.

For a while, I went along acting like everything was okay. I felt numb as I went through the motions of my everyday life and routine. I forced myself to stay calm, managing the household, the kids, and myself as steadily as I could. Protected by my robot like efficiency, I told myself I was fine. I was perfectly capable of handling what had happened.

I had been warned that Marsh needed rest and no stress in order to heal. How could I tell him that I was afraid he would be disabled or die? How could I tell him that I was afraid he would never work again, that I was frozen with anxiety about money for our family's future? How could I tell him that I was infuriated at him for not taking better care of his body and for causing me all this distress? How could I tell him that my trust was eroded, now that he had proved he was not immortal and invincible? How could I tell him how scared I was that he would keel over and die if he was late or missed his pills? How could I tell him that I was waking up in the middle of the night to listen for his breath, scared he was lying dead beside me? How could I tell him that I was afraid to leave the house, sure that his life was my responsibility and that I hated it?

Of course I didn't say these things, at least not aloud to Marsh or to anyone. I was ashamed of my feelings and kept them hidden inside, becoming progressively more isolated and alone. Instead of expressing my fear, I concentrated on my competence. I repaired the back fence with a hammer and nails. I busily painted our bedroom and wallpapered our bathroom. I never once considered how Marsh felt, lying in bed recovering as I frantically painted us into separate corners.

Life became a series of mechanical actions without meaning. Like a coronary artery slowly closing down, the life and love between us got so sluggish it was barely enough to keep our relationship alive.

Months later, I was riding my exercise bicycle when the incongruity of my behavior hit me. Here I was, acting like I didn't need Marsh, when there was no one in the world I treasured more. I was so terrified of losing him that I was pushing him away. Instead of drawing near, I had constructed a wall of bravado between us, trying desperately to prove that I could live without the one person I loved most. After feeling so betrayed, I had been determined never to be that vulnerable again. I had decided that if there was a chance of Marsh's abandoning me, I would leave first: if not physically, then emotionally.

A wave of shame went through me as I realized what I had done. How could I be so selfish? Marsh had been sick and needed me, and I had been concerned only with protecting myself. Like a waterfall, tears began to stream down my face. They washed away my shame, and I forgave myself. Having released the pain, I made a new and conscious vow to share my love and vulnerability, to be Marsh's heartmate.

Acknowledging what exists gives you the raw material for a new start. With acceptance, you can see how the cardiac crisis has affected you. Ventilated anger melts away and new compassion toward your mate and yourself emerges. You can't change what has already happened; neither can you turn back time. But once you've faced reality, grieved, and cleansed your wounds, you can move ahead.

The Power of Images

Trust is based on a series of experiences that provide a reliable image of reality. Whether you're aware of it or not, you probably trust the security of your life-style, a stable relationship with your mate, and your expectations of the future. As each day dawns, and everything you take for granted in your life continues to be there, your images are supported and reinforced. Until something happens to threaten your images, you continue to place your trust in the world view you've created.

Toward the end of *The Great Gatsby*, the narrator wistfully remarks, "It is invariably saddening to look through new eyes at things upon which you have expended your own powers of adjustment."[5] All cardiac spouses share a loss of trust as our images are torn apart by the unexpected shock of heart disease. We need to repair our images to complete the process of healing. In the adult world, images are rarely discussed or taken seriously. Images are considered to be the product of children's imaginations, or of the senility of the aged, or the delusions of the mentally disabled.

Imagery is a combination of our mental and emotional perceptions of events. We believe that the world *is* the way we "see" it. Beyond conscious awareness, our minds and emotions interpret and define reality. Thus our images form the basis of our world view and are the seat of our actions. We trust our images. We respond to them as if they were reality.

If your image of the hospital is of a place with a competent and caring staff, you will feel satisfied with the quality of care your spouse receives. If your image of the hospital is of a place of helplessness and isolation, that may give rise to a very different interpretation: that of an impersonal, untrustworthy place. The truth is probably somewhere in between, but your image is your reality.

The power of imagery and of the mind/matter connection are not well-understood, but even the superstitious are familiar with the concept of a self-fulfilling prophecy: the idea that what we imagine eventually comes to pass. Overhearing the prognosis that his bypass repair was probably "good for five years" may have imprinted an image that had a physical effect on one cardiac patient. Exactly five years later he returned to surgery for a second bypass.

On the positive side, there has been research that indicates that if patients make the effort to construct and then believe positive images, using the technique of visualization to "see" chemicals or rays destroying all the cancer cells in the body, for example, they actually live longer than patients whose imagery is negative.[6]

Programs designed to reverse heart disease are as yet statistically unproven, but cardiac patients who *participate* in their recovery—actively involving themselves in a food plan or exercise program, yoga and meditation, or walking regularly in the local shopping center—and who *believe* that they are promoting their good health, experience an enhanced quality of life. Norman Cousins, author, healer, and heart patient, described walking on a golf course and seeing medics and an ambulance rush to the aid of a man who suddenly collapsed. The medical personnel were monitoring his blood pressure and pulse. Cousins read the monitor, but seeing that the man looked really scared, put his hand on the patient's shoulder, and told him that he had a very strong heart and was going to make it. Within a minute's time the monitor's dangerously high reading had returned almost to normal.[7]

If imagery has power in the physical realm, it seems indisputable that it would affect psychological and spiritual health as well.

Penny, age thirty-two, sat weeping on a park bench as she watched her two toddlers playing enthusiastically on the swings. She was crying because she believed she had lost the potential for what she called a "normal" family. She grieved because her family could not live carelessly or worry-free, now that her husband had heart disease; her children would no longer be innocent offspring of perfectly healthy parents.

In Penny's mind, the image of an ideal family precluded serious illness and pain. Her ability to cry and her willingness to discuss her lost image were encouraging recovery signs. As she worked through her feelings of disappointment and frustration, she began to redefine what "normal" meant, and to rebuild her image of her family's future.

A crisis forces us to focus on what's real. When we hold our images up to that mirror of reality, we get a distorted reflection. Often the pain experienced in a crisis depends on how big a gap looms between what is real and what we wish could be.

Marsh's heart attack changed my image of who my husband really is. I had never given much conscious thought to his mortality. In the life-threatening crisis that brought Marsh to a bed in the coronary care unit, I saw what I had not noticed or thought about until then. Marsh is mortal. That means he will die. Maybe not now, but he won't live forever.

That thought came as a great surprise! I knew that I would die; that realization had come with my mother's death ten years earlier. But I had never applied that to Marsh. My image was of an invincible man. Not only was he physically strong and active, his energy for life had always seemed so unfaltering.

If I thought far enough into the future, to our eighties or nineties, I could imagine us aged and dying. But the day my image was shattered. I was only forty-three.

Marsh was my first love. I "fell for him" when we were in high school. My image of him then was of a handsome blue-eyed blond with an athlete's body, a scholar's mind, an intensity for life, and a powerful moral drive. Had I never looked at him again? Why hadn't I seen the twenty-three years of changes?

The man I saw looking out at me from the tubes, wires, and machinery in the cardiac care unit that night was a half-bald, gray-faced, middle-aged man. Where had my adolescent hero gone? Who was this sick and aging man, his blue eyes flecked with fear and disbelief?

Why had I never noticed time passing? Why had I never brought the image of my mate up to date? My perception of him was unconnected to the real world of the 1980s.

As painful as it was to look time in the face, there was no way to avoid it. Little by little, reminded by my own graying hair and the lines in my face, I began to integrate my image of us, making it more accurate and realistically current. We are no longer teenage lovers, but our lives aren't over by any means. Now my image of us as vital human beings is enriched with the maturity and wisdom that comes with experience.

The pain of hanging on to something that you ought to let go of, or yearning for something that is already gone, can be eased. The cardiac crisis is one of those situations where you must look at your life's old "picture album." Nostalgia is to be expected. And reminiscences about the past can stimulate more good memories and intimacy. But ultimately, your images may need an overhaul. Don't burn the album; see it clearly and then look at today's picture.

You can't always construct images that will keep you safe from pain. An adult cardiac daughter admitted how painful it was to acknowledge that her childhood image of her father was forever lost. She had always carried an image of a powerful and strong Dad. Reality was another story. She witnessed her forceful father, now weak and dependent, requiring a nurse's help to urinate.

The power of one person's images can influence another's. Edy, an earnest woman in her mid-fifties relates, sadly, that her husband, Jake, has been calling himself "damaged goods" ever since his bypass surgery. He is so ashamed that he even suggested that Edy divorce him. Jake's image of himself has so strained their relationship that whenever Edy does anything for him, he accuses her of acting out of pity.

Both Jake and Edy are suffering because Jake has such a limited image of himself. Edy feels helpless, unable to convince Jake that her caring comes from love, and that she doesn't see him as "damaged." Only Jake can transform his image. If he doesn't, it will color his actions, diminish his self-esteem, and may even destroy his relationship with Edy.

In addition to personal images, there are cultural images to cope with. Cultural images influence us because large numbers of people accept them. For example, the great numbers of male cardiac bypass patients help establish an image of acceptance and normalcy. In some cardiac rehabilitation programs the bravado engendered by the cardiac camaraderie even suggests celebrity status. "Zipper chests" are recognized as a badge of courage, and cases are compared and discussed. Conversely, the smaller percentage of women with heart disease suffer with a negative image of disfigurement and isolation. Women lack the "locker room" opportunity for repartée, and are neither prepared nor given support. No one admires their scars or offers suggestions as simple as a front-closing bra, easier to negotiate after bypass surgery.

In general, it doesn't dawn on us to question the accuracy or virtue of cultural images. Some are correct reflections of reality, while others are distorted. It is crucial to question popular misconceptions and images like: Heart disease is a disease of old age; heart disease only affects men; heart disease is caused by high stress; heart disease means the end of normal life—including exercise and all strenuous physical and sexual activity.

Brad, a cardiac spouse in his late fifties, told me how his and Polly's lives were limited by Polly's inaccurate image of herself. Brad first met Polly at a square dance. Although most of their interests were very different, they continued to square dance several times a month over the thirty-five years of their marriage. When Polly had a heart attack, she announced that her square-dancing days were over.

Within a few months, Polly's cardiologist gave her the go-ahead to resume her activities, including dancing, but she was too afraid to consider it. She encouraged Brad to go, but refused to accompany him to the dances, so Brad stayed home.

Square dancing became something that they couldn't talk about; she felt guilty that she had made him give up dancing, and he felt guilty wanting her to go. I asked them to share their worst fear. They both agreed: It was that Polly would suffer another heart attack in the middle of a dance.

Once they had confronted their most terrifying image, their fear lost some of its power. They decided to go to the next weekend dance. Brad reported how excited and scared they were. Brad danced the entire evening. Polly alternated between dancing and sitting out. They went home early, exhilarated and exhausted. But they had a wonderful time, reminiscing about the night they first met, discovering how happy they were to still have each other and dance, too.

Your own self-image can limit or free you. Start now to *redefine* and *update* your images of yourself and your mate. Bring your images up to date, let go of the past, and live more fully in the present.

Updating Your Images

The nature of your reality is forever different because of the cardiac crisis. Acknowledging that the images you relied on are broken leaves you confused. The old image no longer fits, but you have yet to create a new one. You may understand intellectually that the image you had was inaccurate, but now what? What can you believe in? Where will you find new images that reflect reality more accurately? How can you create images for your new attitudes and actions?

Mending your broken images requires a courageous look; a clear assessment of the accuracy of your images as compared to an objective reality; the strength to let go of anything inaccurate, outdated, or self-destructive; and a conscious effort to replace the old images with newer, healthier, more appropriate ones.

Here is a Heartmates® exercise designed to help you examine the images that presently motivate or direct your life. Use each set of questions as a guide. Respond with both your head and your heart. Don't be concerned about writing full sentences, making sense, or being logical. Use these questions to explore your images as fully as you can.

HEARTMATES® GUIDE FOR EXAMINING IMAGES

1. *What do you recall about first visiting your mate in the hospital?* See your mate and the coronary care unit as a still photo; then add sounds, smells, and movement to your image. What nonverbal message did you receive about your spouse's condition? In your mind's eye, see yourself then; what were you feeling, thinking, doing? Describe your communication, feelings, level of intimacy with your mate.

2. *Create an image of your mate's physical heart.* As much as you can, visualize the actual damage as well as its symbolic meaning. Then see the healing that has occurred. How is your mate's physical and emotional heart different now than before the onset of heart disease? Based on your image, how do you envision the long-term quality of your mate's life? Imagine yourself five years and then ten years into the future. What effects has your mate's heart disease had on your life? How do you expect the picture will continue to change?

3. *What image of home and family do you have from the period of active recovery?* What concerns did you have then about caring for your mate, your family, yourself? See in your mind's eye the network of communication and feelings that connected your family then. How was the family different during recovery than before the

cardiac crisis? What is your image of your family now? As you see your family at present, note what issues your family is dealing with and what is going well for all of you.

4. *Look into a mirror of your past. Who were you before your mate's heart crisis?* What was important to you? What was your relationship with your mate like? How was your daily life organized? What were your priorities? How did you define your purpose for living? Gather this past image of you and set it aside.

5. *Stand in front of the same mirror right now. Who are you today?* What do you know about your strengths and limitations? How do you feel about yourself now? What is important to you today? What is your relationship with your mate like? How do you organize your daily life? What are your priorities? What is your purpose for living? Gather this present image of you and put it alongside your past image.

6. *Step back far enough to be able to see both images in the mirror.* Visualize how being a cardiac spouse has changed you. What have you learned? How have you weathered the changes? How would you assess your acceptance of what's happened to you? Have you forgiven your mate, yourself? Are you taking care of your most important needs? Are you continuing to mourn your losses and heal your wounds?

Purposeful examination of our images allows us to update them continually as time passes and conditions change. One of the advantages of taking stock and comparing past and present images is that you can appreciate new qualities you've developed in yourself as a response to the cardiac crisis. Claire, who had always described herself as someone "without a head for figures," took over the family finances when her husband, Tim, was hospitalized because of a heart attack. Tim had always paid the bills, balanced the family checkbook, and made the financial decisions. Claire, busy with her handicrafts and weaving, was glad to let Tim handle that aspect of their life; she wasn't interested and believed she was incompetent with numbers.

After four months of being the family banker, Claire confessed that she enjoyed keeping the books. She discovered that the more she worked with figures, the more her confidence grew. Tim congratulated her for being a "crack book-keeper." Claire occasionally regressed and thought of herself in the old way, but when she told Tim this, he just laughed in retrospect at all the years she had never even subtracted her checks in the checkbook.

Recognizing your outdated images will help you disengage yourself from them. If you can catch yourself falling back on old images, you can learn to stop. Your mate may be willing to keep an eye out for behavior akin to your old images, so he can point out when you've limited yourself. Then you can consciously replace the old image with a new one that is more realistic and up-to-date.

What do you want your new images to be? What qualities do you want to develop? Some qualities a cardiac spouse could use are: clarity, wisdom, love, strength, gratitude, humor, and forgiveness. Write the quality you desire most in large letters on a three-by-five-inch card. Place the card where you will see it often, where it will attract your attention. The refrigerator door and the mirror above my bathroom sink are my favorite places. Look at the word each day to keep the image active in your mind, even when you aren't paying conscious attention. Visualize how you can express the quality in your daily life. When you stop noticing the card, move it to your bedside, or make a new different colored card with different shaped letters to attract your attention. Keep that reminder in view.

• • •

SOME IDEAS TO REMEMBER ABOUT IMAGES

• Everyone has images.
• People experience their images differently: some people summon visual pictures; others "sense" their images.
• People respond to images as if they were reality.
• Images influence understanding, attitudes, and actions.
• Images can affect physical and emotional health.
• Creating new images requires conscious effort.
• Lost images need to be mourned.
• Defining yourself by an outdated image limits who you are and what you can do. Update your images and free yourself.

Forgiveness

The final step in the healing process is forgiveness. Mentally chastising yourself for your feelings clogs the process and impedes healing. Once you can understand and accept what has happened, you will be able to be compassionate and forgiving.

One cardiac spouse, Betsy, has spent most of her time since Jeff's surgery berating herself for being angry. Even though she "knew" she should be grateful for Jeff's recovery, she couldn't stop feeling sorry for herself. The more she tried to be solicitous, covering her anger and pretending to be concerned only about Jeff, the more resentful she became. She was hurt that no one recognized or appreciated her pain despite the fact that she kept it to herself.

When Betsy was able to recognize that she was responsible for keeping herself isolated, the process of forgiveness began. As her defenses crumbled, Betsy was able to release her feelings and understand that she too had been wounded. Being gentle and forgiving toward herself also set the stage for her to be able to forgive Jeff.

When you get a sense of your mate's and your own mortality, your life comes into sharp focus. Forgiveness is motivated by the human longing for reconciliation. When there are fractures in relationships and unaccepted grievances, reconciliation can heal. The urge, given the acknowledgment of mortality, to "finish business" and clean up relationships, is at the core of forgiveness.

Forgiveness usually demands a transformation in attitude. Reluctance to give up a grievance may be the result of pride, stubbornness, or fear of rejection. If you are willing to apologize and make amends, you're already making a new start. The anxiety of strained relationships and wounded psyches is ameliorated by forgiveness, a step on the journey to inner peace.

The cardiac patient and the cardiac spouse need to forgive the imperfection implied by heart disease. The illusion of perfection often crumbles with the onset of the cardiac crisis. Many heart patients experience deep anger at their bodies' betrayal; some go as far as to consider divorce to punish themselves or to protect their spouses from having to live with "second-best."

Believing that you are worthwhile and deserve love just because you are human, not because you are perfect, is a major shift in thinking that requires real psychological effort. You need to accept and forgive your mate for his imperfections, including heart disease. Equally important, you need to accept and forgive yourself and God.

Sources of Support

No one can heal all alone. You need and deserve support and encouragement to get through your grief.

Physical Support. When you use so much of your vital and emotional energy to grieve, you need to pay special attention to your physical care. Take extra vitamins. Avoid physical excesses. Be sure you get the extra sleep you need. Eat nutritious and good-tasting food regularly. Drink six-eight glasses of water every day. Wear clothes that are comfortable, cozy, and warm. Take a walk every day or stick to your regular fitness plan, but remember that this is not the time to start a strenuous, new exercise program. If possible, arrange to have a regular therapeutic massage. See your physician for any physical symptoms of stress. If you question a specific activity, ask yourself, "Will this help me focus on my feelings?" This is not indulgent, it is essential for you to concentrate on your needs and keep your physical maintenance at a simple, stable level.

Emotional support. Here are some things you can do to support yourself emotionally. Listen to music that you find beautiful and harmonic. Treat yourself to soothing teas and favorite foods. Pamper yourself. Invite help from family and friends when you feel overwhelmed. Share your feelings with a trusted confidante. Stay away from places, people, and activities that are harsh or cold or overly demanding. Think of positive memories that evoke your feelings of pleasure and gratitude. Laugh aloud every day. If you have no one available, seek emotional support from a therapist or grief counselor. Grief groups and support groups may meet at your hospital, your church, or your local community center.

Spiritual Support. Many people find their spirits replenished in nature. Breathe deeply and inhale fresh air in your city park or along a country road to revitalize yourself. Nothing feels more nurturing than the warmth of the sun in the sky overhead and the security of the earth under your feet. Gardening has beneficial effects. Water is also healing to the spirit; take warm baths and frequent showers. Walk by your favorite lake or, if it's near, enjoy the ocean's sound and spray.

It may be that the cardiac crisis has reawakened or deepened your religious connection. By accepting your limitations and turning to a greater source, your spirit will be nourished. Many people find that religious services and familiar rituals offer peace. Some may be comforted just sitting in a silent chapel. Others find profound value in prayer or meditation. Talk to your minister, priest, rabbi, or a spiritual leader. You know best what will help you. Make a commitment to support your spiritual self.

Turning Toward the Future

Time alone isn't enough to heal all wounds. But with the courage to face your pain and the willingness to update your images, active mourning does end! There are clues that you have grieved enough. You can mark your progress by the fact that life has started to return to "normal." As you reorient yourself from the past into the present, more realistic images signal that you are healing.

One strong sign of recovery is commonly described as "a sense of release." A cardiac spouse realized her new freedom when whole days went by without her thinking about her spouse's heart condition or wishing for life as it used to be. Another woman was delighted when she became aware that she was beginning to look ahead. She confidently made plane reservations for next winter's family vacation.

Spontaneous and genuine interest in others is an important indication that the cardiac crisis is behind you. I remember with pleasure the cardiac spouse who remarked enthusiastically of "finally being released from the prison of my own pain." In the year since her husband's surgery, she had been so involved that she was barely able to tolerate conversation on anything other than her spouse's condition. Her world seemed to open like a flower as she anticipated spending meaningful time with friends and family again.

Another characteristic of healing is "renewed energy." During the acute crisis and often in the long months of recovery, most of your vital energy was expended just to get through each day. Fatigue and exhaustion were common complaints. Now, gradually (or sometimes in a dramatic burst) you gain enough physical strength to do things that for months you've been unable to consider, let alone accomplish. You'll have renewed emotional energy; you may *want* to plant a garden, make plans with friends, and participate in leisure activities with or without your mate. You might pick up a stimulating novel or involve yourself in a new project.

That you can now make better judgments is another sign of your recovery. Of course, circumstances necessitated your making serious decisions long before this time, but the difference is qualitative. Recall how consuming and exhausting it felt to make decisions. Remember your confusion and frustration when you couldn't think things through? Now your ability to concentrate without undue effort has returned. Once again you can follow through fully and efficiently.

The return of regular eating habits and pre-crisis sleeping patterns, the easiest signs to measure, may be the last to occur. Things will change gradually, until the present has integrated both the lessons of the past and your hopes for the future.

Re-pairing the
Heartmate Connection

*T*he marriage bond, symbolized by the heart in song and literature, has been threatened by the cardiac crisis. Your connection was first broken during your spouse's stay in the hospital. Once he returned home, each of you remained isolated as you tried to protect each other from undue stress.

Heart disease affects *all* relationships, including strong, loving ones. According to author and social scientist Edward J. Speedling, when a physical trauma of the magnitude of a cardiac crisis occurs, the marital relationship is challenged. "The act of healing cannot be complete until the social and emotional bonds which the illness disrupted are revitalized."[1]

The cardiac crisis draws some couples closer together, resulting in greater intimacy and support. Many heartmates' devotion to each other is enhanced. You may have become acutely aware of how much you cherish and need your mate. For other cardiac couples, the trauma pulls them apart, intensifying already existing conflicts. You may now see even more clearly the flaws in your relationship.

Unfortunately, for a few, the cardiac crisis is the final rift in an already estranged relationship.

It's not fair to blame all the imperfections in your marriage on heart disease. The patterns of your relationship were established long ago. And yet, without a doubt, the cardiac crisis has had a powerful effect. Conversely, the quality of your marriage has affected your physical and emotional recovery.

A relationship requires two partners. It's a mistake to assume that once the patient has recovered physically, the marriage is automatically healed. In order for the relationship to mend, you and your mate need to recover individually and put effort into healing the relationship. At the very least, a relationship needs to be flexible enough to adapt to a new reality which includes heart disease.

The cardiac crisis can be the catalyst for a more intimate relationship. Repairing the heartmate connection is the final stage in your recovery. Honest confrontation of the changes in your relationship is a step toward deepening the marriage connection.

Communication Between Heartmates

The value of good communication is generally recognized in our society. The cardiac crisis has undoubtedly had an impact on your communication patterns. For some couples, the disruption is minor, like assuming a quieter tone of voice. For others, more dramatic changes range from an overly polite stance to no communication at all.

Caring communication is essential for healing a wounded relationship. If you sense that the cardiac crisis has strained the communication in your relationship, speak up! As hard as it sounds, if you can break the forbidding silence or shift your conversation from safe subjects to more personal topics you will most effectively improve the situation. You must first look honestly at the changes.

One way to assess change is to determine how your present communication differs from that before the cardiac crisis. Use this checklist to help you evaluate your present communication with your mate. (As you answer the questions, keep in mind how you would have responded before the crisis.)

HEARTMATES® COMMUNICATION EVALUATION CHECKLIST

Yes   *No*

_____ _____ 1. Has your tone of voice or the way you talk to your mate changed?

_____ _____ 2. Are you careful about the words you use when you talk to your mate?

_____ _____ 3. Are there long silences when just the two of you are together?

_____ 4. Is it difficult to keep conversation going between you?

_____ 5. Do you direct conversation away from yourselves and toward others?

_____ 6. Is your television on more than before the cardiac crisis?

_____ _____ 7. Are you less expressive of your feelings?

_____ _____ 8. Are you more silent about your concerns?

_____ _____ 9. Do you feel more lonely, isolated, stuck?

_____ _____ 10. Do you talk regularly about daily and long-term plans and dreams?

_____ _____ 11. Do you have permission to discuss "taboo" issues (life and death, sex, finances, love) since the cardiac crisis?

_____ _____ 12. Are you generally satisfied and emotionally supported by the communication you have with your mate?

A comparison of communication before and after can be useful; however, some people find it difficult to be objective and concrete about their lives. Visualization is another, more abstract way to assess changes in communication. Imagine the heartmate bond as a cord that connects you and your mate. Picture, for a moment, the symbolic flow of communication between your two hearts. How much moves through the cord? What color is the substance? Is it thick or thin, sticky or flowing smoothly? Is the passageway tight and clogged, or is the cord clean and open to the flow of communication?

This exercise can help you to see your modes of communication more clearly. If your answers reveal major changes in communication, ask yourself if these are positive or negative. The same is true for the image you summon: does it evoke a picture of the communication flow opened, severed, or somewhere in between? For some couples, the cardiac crisis provokes very serious soul-searching and sharing. Other couples become self-conscious and estranged, and, in the most extreme cases, live like strangers.

Myths to Dispel

The way you communicate is further influenced by myths. A myth is a culturally learned belief that affects your emotions and actions. As a cardiac spouse, you are vulnerable to three myths.

Myth 1. *It is better for the patient if you don't communicate your concerns or fears.* Protection is the idea underlying this myth. When your mate was in the hospital, rules limiting visiting hours were faithfully observed to ensure his rest. There was no way to prevent your private communication from being public. When you were allowed to visit, your time was short, and often interrupted by staff continuing the regimen of physical care.

The loss of unlimited privacy translates into the attitude that it's best just to reassure the patient with a smile, a kiss, and casual conversation. And many couples feel inhibited about expressing their affection in front of others.

As a rule, cardiac spouses believe that it's best not to worry the patient with concerns of any kind. One woman proudly announced that she was taking such good care of her hospitalized husband that he had no inkling she had taken a job to meet their medical expenses. Another cardiac spouse struggled alone with her teenage son's drinking problem, rather than solicit his father's involvement in making difficult and important decisions.

Your love for your mate, coupled with a culturally ingrained myth, is a powerful motivation to protect him. But it's a mistake to conceal your concern. Heart patients, men and women alike, lie in hospital beds worrying about the same things as their spouses. Your spouse is probably grappling with fears of dying, being disabled, and failing to provide for your family. Heart patients confront serious questions: Why do I have heart disease? Why did I survive? Will you still love me? Does this mean I'll die young, without seeing my children grown or my grandchildren born?

Avoiding communication about these important concerns only maintains distance. It neither alleviates the concerns nor heals the communication breakdown. Continuing to withhold feelings intensifies the isolation each of you feels. If your spouse hides having chest pain, and if you don't reveal your fears and doubts, the chasm between you will grow. Sometimes even information-bearing communication is cut off when you are estranged by the cardiac crisis. If it is too threatening to begin discussing feelings, stick to the daily concerns each of you has until you become more comfortable talking together. Decide together whether you should continue plans to redo the kitchen, where you might take your vacation, how you can help your child with his college expenses. Ask your mate where the deed to the house is located, or begin to explore the financial details of his retirement plan at work. Suggest that it would be wise to inform your children of the whereabouts of your wills and insurance policies. These topics are preliminary information for future planning for the two of you to do together.

There is no proof that avoiding communication is beneficial to a heart patient, and holding back increases your feelings of loneliness and abandonment. The relationship itself weakens without quality communication.

Myth 2. *Stress is reduced by withholding anger and other negative feelings.* If you believe that silence relieves stress, you may withhold your feelings. However, the exact opposite is true. Stress increases, not decreases, when we consciously withhold our emotions. Sharing them allows you to honestly let go of fear, guilt, and anger.

Communication gets stifled by withheld anger. If you bite your tongue, silently clench your fists, and replace honest feelings with bitterness or barbs, you may be camouflaging unexpressed anger. Dr. Theodore Rubin asserts that expressing anger can actually strengthen a relationship.[2] He contends that expressing anger demonstrates that a spouse cares enough to want more intimacy and is willing to invest emotional energy in the relationship. Showing your spouse your feelings requires courage because it makes you vulnerable. It is also a statement of confidence that your relationship can withstand difficulties and disagreement, and will emerge strengthened by the experience.

Ask yourself when was the last time you and your mate spoke angrily to each other. And lovingly? If it's been a while, make a commitment to start talking. Be generous in your expectations of yourself. The longer it's been since you've disclosed your feelings, the more you will need to ease back into sharing your feelings. Begin by taking small steps.

Myth 3. *Good communication means agreement.* Remember, as you make tentative communication, that everyone prefers agreement. Wouldn't it be nice if you told your mate that you felt angry and hurt that he no longer seemed interested in your work, and his response was: "I'm in total agreement with you. You're absolutely right." While most of us would like to avoid conflict, *people do disagree.* Disagreement is a healthy part of a relationship. If you and your spouse agreed about everything, your life together would be rather boring. You might as well have married a mirror.

Making decisions together often accentuates differences. Divergent ways of coping with a crisis can create tension and put additional stress on a relationship. Ronald and Tina had difficulty making a decision about his surgery. When his cardiologist recommended a bypass operation, Ronald wanted to schedule it immediately. In her usual inquisitive style, Tina continued to ask questions, suggested getting a second opinion, and was generally opposed to Ronald checking into the hospital immediately. Ron felt anxious and felt a lack of support from Tina, while Tina said she just couldn't say "yes" when she needed more information and time to get used to the idea. Ron responded by refusing to consult with another doctor. Tina tried to throw the whole decision on Ron, believing that if the surgery turned out less than perfect, it would be all his fault. Without the help of a close friend, they might not have been able to discuss their differences. Expressing their fears and their need for each other's love enabled them to understand their differences and reach a decision they both supported.

Learning to tolerate your mate's differences is crucial for communication. Good communication requires more than just thoughtless talking and listening. It is the process of making and maintaining contact with another person.

Loving contact and clear communication are more difficult in a time of crisis. Be gentle with yourself and your heartmate as you try to improve your communication. Keep your expectations realistic, and celebrate your successes together.

Here are some "do's" and "don'ts" to help you and your mate improve communication.

HEARTMATES® COMMUNICATION GUIDELINES

DO	DON'T
Do say how you feel	Don't withdraw for fear you'll stress your mate
Do remember that your spouse has similar concerns	Don't believe the myth that communication is harmful
Do express your anger	Don't believe your relationship is too fragile to bear your feelings
Do try to understand differences between you and your mate	Don't be scared off by your mate's individual style of expression
Do respect your own needs	Don't forget that unspoken feelings ooze out indirectly
Do focus on loving each other	Don't avoid talking about important concerns

DO	DON'T
Do enlist help from a friend if you reach an impasse	Don't forget that communication can be difficult
Do honor individual differences	Don't mistake disagreement for disapproval

Sexuality and the Cardiac Relationship

Cardiac spouses of all ages have been affected by the sexual revolution of the 1960s. Following the publication of the Kinsey Report, people began to talk more openly about their sexuality. What before had been taboo was considered legitimate subject matter for scientific research. Despite these gains, it is still true that "nice" people don't talk about sex, at least "nice" people over the age of thirty.

For many people in your age bracket, the cardiac crisis may be the first time that you explore and discuss sexual issues. Propriety and etiquette are less important as you consider what really matters in your life. *This is a time when we both deeply need and strongly fear being connected sexually with each other.* The cardiac crisis provides the opportunity for us to talk about our sexuality and cultivate sexual expression with our mates.

Both men and women still have difficulty accepting their bodies. Your images about sexuality originated with parents, teachers, religious authorities, and the media. Examining your values can give you new insight into your attitudes and behavior. One cardiac spouse put it beautifully when she said, "I was never very satisfied with my body as a young woman. Now, in my fifties, I'm just beginning to discover that my body is a source of pleasure and comfort."

Not so long ago, men and women both believed that sex was something that men enjoyed and women put up with. The sexual revolution was influential in disproving that fallacy. Still, few people describe their sexual expression as a source of profound satisfaction and fulfillment.

Decades after the sexual revolution, it is still rare for medical professionals to initiate a personal discussion or actively solicit a cardiac couple's questions about the sexual aspect of their relationship. Sometimes you can find a copy of the American Heart Association's 1983 pamphlet called "Sex and Heart Disease" at your hospital or in the waiting room of your cardiac rehabilitation facility. Often, coronary care units include sex education as a part of their overall educational service for cardiac patients and spouses. But sex is still so sensitive and personal an issue that it is difficult for some professionals to be really helpful.

Only days after Marsh's heart attack, just before his release, a nurse brought a portable tape recorder and a tape to his room for us. It was a tape about sexuality and heart disease.

A strange voice came out of the machine telling me, "It was a good sign that my husband was feeling well enough to notice how attractive the nurses' legs looked." That made me angry. I wanted to scream at the voice in the immobile blue machine on the window sill, "How could you understand? I don't care if we ever have intercourse again. I'm terrified that he's going to die." Sex was the last thing on my mind a mere week after his heart attack. And I thought the tape was impersonal and offensive.

We laughed sort of self-consciously together and turned it off. I felt misunderstood and wondered if my concern about sex, or lack of concern, were unusual.

When Marsh came home and we were going to sleep together in our own bed, he put his arms around me and I fell asleep feeling secure and comforted. For some weeks sex was not a high priority.

When I did begin to think about it, my fears were overwhelming. I heard echoes from the portable tape recorder but they didn't diminish my terror. Marsh might die from the stress or excitement of an orgasm. Or maybe, at forty-three, my sex life as I had known it was over; perhaps

Marsh was impotent, a side effect of his drugs. Or maybe he was disinterested because he had heart disease. Not so young and liberated that I could directly ask him about it, I kept my fear quiet, not sure how to broach the subject without humiliating Marsh and embarrassing myself.

All cardiac couples have questions about sex. There isn't anyone, regardless of any level of confidence, who doesn't have some anxiety about how heart disease will affect the sexual relationship.

There are five main *misconceptions* surrounding the subject of sex and heart disease. Each one contributes to feelings of fear and apprehension. They are:

1. Sexual activity is hazardous for heart patients.
2. Heart disease decreases libido and impairs sexual functioning.
3. Heart disease signifies the end of normal sexual activity.
4. Sexual prowess is the measure of masculinity, and masculinity is the measure of a male's human worth.
5. Sex is love.

None of these is true. Replace them with the truth. If you're like most cardiac spouses, you have other concerns, too. Your most pressing fear may be that your sexual relationship will be permanently damaged, destroying the closeness in your marriage. This is an absolutely natural fear, particularly in the beginning stages of recovery, which are like the first weeks after having a baby, when couples are advised to postpone sexual relations.

The early recommendation to abstain may give you the false idea that your sexual relationship is over. Although it takes some time, *the overwhelming majority of cardiac couples are able to resume their previous sexual relationship.*

It is generally accepted that cardiac patients experience a temporary decrease in sexual drive. There are three main reasons for the decline in libido: physical fatigue, depression, and side effects from medications. All of these factors can be treated, and usually dissipate over time.

Knowing that "this too will pass" doesn't necessarily lessen your fear. People in crisis also need information to help set their fears to rest. To get beyond the misconceptions, we need to examine the most current medical facts about the physical aspects of sexual activity.

Cardiac couples are fortunate because there *are* answers available, at least about male heart patients. There is yet to be a study dealing with the sexual needs, habits, and behavior of female cardiac patients, although women make up a growing percentage of the cardiac population.

In an article printed in the Harvard Medical School Health Letter, Dr. Thomas Hackett, Chief of Psychiatry at Massachusetts General Hospital and Professor of Psychiatry at Harvard Medical School, addresses many of the questions about sex raised by male heart patients and their spouses.[3]

According to Hackett, the depression that commonly follows a heart attack includes reduced feelings of sexual desire. In addition, patients in active recovery are easily fatigued and spend lots of time alone, reflecting on what has happened to them. Natural depression from trauma to the body diminishes desire. Hackett points out that for 85 percent of patients this depression (and related reduced libido) passes and never becomes a major problem. If, after three months, impotence continues, treatment is recommended.

"There appears to be no medical basis for implicating satisfying sex, in a familiar and supportive relationship, as a hazard."[4] Research done with cardiac couples who had stable, long-term relationships documented that the average amount of energy expended while having sex is equivalent to climbing one flight of stairs. To reduce your fear, watch your mate climb a flight of stairs. (I suggest you let

that information sink in, and not have intercourse immediately following his climb!)

Like other physical activity, sexual participation
should be resumed gradually during recovery. Dr. Hackett
advises that a cardiac couple limit themselves to foreplay
and abstain from intercourse for the first two to three
weeks of recovery. He stresses that this is "not because it's
dangerous but because it takes the pressure off both partners to perform. Masturbation is also perfectly safe and
may ease the transition back to partnered sex. After three
weeks there are usually no restrictions, though this schedule may be modified in cases of severe illness."[5]

The fear of dying during intercourse should not be
dismissed summarily, or without additional information. A
Japanese study analyzing the cause of 5,000 sudden deaths
found that of those, 34 died (presumably) during intercourse. Of those, 30 were with partners other than their
own spouses. And virtually all had blood levels close to, or
in the range of, intoxication. This data suggests that the
lethal stress was not the act of intercourse, but that intercourse in combination with alcohol and in the context of an
extramarital affair may be hazardous.

Some medications used to lower blood pressure,
prevent palpitations, or control angina may, as a side effect,
diminish libido or produce impotence. Drugs may affect
female cardiac patients as well by reducing natural lubrica-
tion. Work with your physician to find medications that
don't have these side effects. Because of reticence on the
part of professionals, it is important that the two of you be
able to discuss the issue and raise it with your physician,
and that you persist until you get the answers and results
you seek.

Jean, a seventy-five-year-old cardiac spouse, recalled a visit with her doctor twenty-five years ago. Usually
reserved and embarrassed, Jean mustered her courage to
ask him about sex. She told her physician that she and her

husband had been turning their backs in bed to avoid arousing each other. Both were afraid that sexual activity would endanger his life. Their doctor emphatically informed Jean that there was no physical risk and that they could safely resume. At seventy-five, Jean whispered shyly that it had made their last years together more precious.

Information helps us dismiss the myths. The vast majority of patients can and do return to normal sex lives within three months of the cardiac event. The physical position adopted in intercourse appears to make no difference in the amount of stress of the sexual activity. There is no medical basis to support one sexual position being safer than another, although many cardiac couples automatically switch to female superior position with the male underneath, thinking that a more passive posture will be less stressful.

Your comfort and confidence is far more important than your choice of positions. Falling back on what you're used to is less stressful than trying to learn new ways of being sexual right now.

If there is a problem with erection, medications should be checked. And, of course, if severe depression and/or specific sexual difficulties continue for longer than several months, consult with your physician.

Sexuality and Self-image

It is natural for recovering male heart patients, who are coping with a changing self-image, to question their virility. The notion that masculinity is measured by sexual prowess sorely needs revision. This misconception affects male cardiac patients of all ages, adding unnecessary pressure to their physical and emotional recovery.

Hospitalized heart patients fear they are dying. Their real concerns about sexuality only begin once they feel confident about surviving. Cardiac patients who flirt with young nurses are most likely experiencing shock and denial. Nurses who respond to sexual talk at face value fail to understand the fear and insecurity resting just below the surface.

Some cardiac couples return to "normal" sexual activity as though nothing has happened. Sex, used as proof that "everything's fine," is only a temporary cover-up. It's confusing, when both of you know that things aren't "fine" or "just like they used to be," to pretend that everything is the same. A frank discussion of sex breaks through that destructive pretense.

Cardiac patients either joke or refer to themselves as "damaged goods." This usually reflects a fear of impotence or of being unable to perform like a "whole" man. If this is the case, you may hesitate to encourage your husband to return to sexual activity for fear of adding to his feelings of inadequacy. However, avoiding intimacy will only intensify the problem, and keep you both from taking that difficult but necessary step back toward a healthy sexual relationship.

As a cardiac spouse, you too may be forced to cope with a changing self-image that affects your sexuality. A full year into recovery, one forty-nine-year-old wife of a bypass patient complained that she couldn't quite bring herself to be sexual very often. Although she didn't entirely understand why, she carried around an uneasy feeling that both she and her husband had suddenly gone from being young and attractive to being "over the hill." Another woman, terrified that her husband would have a heart attack in her arms, maintained a separate bedroom and refused to sleep with him at all.

Recovery may temporarily inhibit your sex life. But heart disease may not be the only factor to consider. Whether or not you have noticed, the frequency and style of your sexual relationship has changed gradually over the years. Some natural decline in frequency of intercourse is documented in people after the age of forty. The cardiac crisis may accelerate that change or bring the decline into focus.

It's unrealistic to try to maintain a standard that was established in your twenties and thirties. Television suggests that youth and speed are what counts, contributing to the pressure to perform. But maturity and comfort are equally valuable. Over time I have become accustomed to Marsh's habit of nodding off during the ten o'clock news, and, let's face it, I'm no longer able to be focused, witty, or romantic at midnight. But I relish and appreciate the softer, quieter, and more vulnerable way we embrace.

Beyond Facts About Sexuality

Facts and information help, but they're no substitute for discussion. Be honest with your need for intimacy. It's essential. Here, as in other areas of your relationship, you will find that you and your mate differ, sometimes significantly and other times in minor ways. One of you may be eager to resume a sexual relationship, while the other may be more reticent. Be patient and kind with each other. Each of you has expectations and fears that need to be acknowledged and aired.

You are separate individuals *and* you are allies, members of the same team. Being teammates is especially essential when it comes to something so sensitive as sex. The cardiac crisis provides the opportunity to examine your changing sexual intimacy in a way that gradual aging doesn't. And for many couples, the imposed hiatus is a chance to appreciate each other and see with new eyes.

Right now, both of you need to give and receive physical comfort. Most couples are able eventually to return to pre-crisis sexual activity. In the great majority of cases, there is no medical contraindication to doing so. As time passes, changes in your mate's physical health may require further adjustments. If the severity of your mate's heart disease results in your being unable to have intercourse, it is a real loss, and one you can grieve over together. If you avoid the pain or deny the need for physical intimacy and don't talk about it, your chances of turning to new, less strenuous ways of being with each other sexually are greatly diminished. In the wake of a crisis, it takes conscious effort, and some creativity, to face what is lost and find new ways to replace it.

Your sexual needs may be in flux along with other changing values and priorities. Perhaps you can be more openly appreciative of each other's affection, more direct about your needs, and more willing to give. With or without heart disease, none of us knows how long we have to live a satisfying life. If you express your love today, and you find yourself together tomorrow, you are blessed with more opportunity to live and love.

Many cardiac couples find themselves closer after the cardiac crisis than during any other period in their relationship. However, it is not unusual for cardiac spouses to confront an emotional barrier of unexpressed fear, resentment, or anger. It's hard to "make love" before those feelings are released and forgiven. Some people hold back, fearful of depending on their mates. Vulnerability motivates others to work harder on their relationships. The threat of loss may ultimately open your hearts to each other. Petty irritations and aggravating differences may seem unimportant in the light of the bond heart disease has threatened.

Most couples find themselves uneasy discussing sexuality in the best of times, even when their relationship is solid and stable. A richer relationship demands the courage of both partners to talk openly about sex. Begin little by little. Tell your heartmate how wonderful it is to be held close, how much you missed the normal contact of sleeping together. Talk about your expectations and desires. There are so many ways to be intimate. Just holding hands or embracing can be enough to express caring physically. Saying "I love you" goes a long way, too.

Once you've opened up about your feelings, begin to discuss your differences respectfully and lovingly. Discuss resolutions that take both of your needs into account. Make a date to give or get a back rub, to cuddle, or to have intercourse. Scheduling time together is a way to say that your relationship is a special priority in your lives. Communication doesn't solve all problems, but conflicts and unmet needs hidden in the back of your mind can grow out of proportion. Ask each other for what you want and need. It can relieve the anguish of sexual expectations and performance anxiety.

One last misconception to debunk is the idea that sex is love. Sex is not love, although it is often mistaken for it. Cardiac couples can adapt to changes in sexual expression more easily if they have faith in the love that bonds them together. Love is experienced in many ways. Physical expressions: a touch, a kiss, a caress, sexual intercourse, are just parts of the repertoire human beings have to express themselves.

Sexual activity is more than sport, pleasure, or comfort. On a deeper level, it can be a way to fully experience yourself and transcend a given moment of time. Sex is at once the most distorted and violated, yet potentially sacred and beautiful of spiritual and physical acts. As you heal your relationship together, give sexual intercourse its correct value in your life. Do not under or over estimate its worth. Your connection to each other needs revitalization and support in order to heal. Your sexual relationship is a symbol of your love and your union. It is a way to celebrate life and your bond as heartmates.

Healing the Heartmate Relationship

Constructive and creative change requires your willingness to examine your relationship, the vulnerability to hope for increased intimacy, the compassion to forgive each other for past disappointments, and the persistence to plan and carry out the small, everyday rearrangements. You must renew your commitment to your relationship.

Sadly, there are those for whom the cardiac crisis is the event which precipitates a final breakdown of the relationship. Gloria, a forty-nine-year-old cardiac spouse, described how she and her fifty-three-year-old husband, Bill, were considering a legal separation after sixteen years of marriage when Bill suffered a heart attack. Months of recovery passed; Bill's response to his disease was irritability and anger directed at Gloria. Her dilemma was a "catch-22." It had been difficult enough, for all the usual reasons, to consider divorce. Could she create a new life for herself? Where would she find support when most of her family and friends were married and loyal to them as a couple? Their marriage was no longer right. But now, with Bill's heart attack, Gloria was afraid of being cast as a selfish, irresponsible person turning her back on a sick man, like a captain abandoning a sinking ship.

No one would advise a couple to separate or divorce during recovery, because of the additional stress. Yet there are relationships that cannot be healed. Usually in these extreme cases, one or both partners have given up hope and are unwilling to put any more effort and good will into the relationship. It is wise to seek professional help in such a situation to provide both of you the support and guidance you'll need to work through this major life crisis.

One of the most important elements of any healing relationship is rebuilding the trust that was shattered. The fear of being abandoned is a fundamental one all human beings live with. Cardiac spouses react in a variety of ways, from being overprotective to feigning fierce independence. Acknowledging your fear, at first to yourself and than to your mate, is a prerequisite for healing the trust between you. Your mate can't realistically guarantee that he'll be there for you—forever. That alone is difficult and painful to admit. But once you can accept that there is no guarantee, you can begin anew, planning for a future which will include an appreciation of the ephemeral nature of life.

Whatever the state of your relationship, your challenge is to see the reality and make peace with it. Only then is there the opportunity to take advantage of new perception and understanding, and to reconnect at a level based on mutual appreciation and respect. Your marriage bond may be strengthened by sharing and surviving this experience together.

As serious and significant as your relationship is, nothing is a more powerful healer than humor. Being able to laugh at yourselves and your situation will help you see things as they truly are and enjoy your togetherness.

One of the best investments we made when Marsh was recovering from bypass surgery was a VCR. Funny movies helped us pass many hours of recuperation, but more significant, the films gave us something to laugh about, together. Marsh complained when he aggravated his incision pain by laughing too hard, but we both found it healing.

Finally, repairing the heartmate connection depends on how well the balance between the individuals needs and relationship needs can be negotiated. A healthy relationship requires each partner to establish and protect individuality and simultaneously reach beyond that to care about each other. This *is the most difficult challenge you face*. The cardiac crisis has made you more aware of your needs. Individual integrity means protecting your best self. Loving your mate means truly supporting and being there for him. Sometimes it's hard to see what's best. More often, it is difficult to determine how you can act in a way that honors both of you and the relationship. The wisdom of all recovery programs is to focus on one day at a time. Healing your relationship requires ongoing commitment, honesty, and love.

> When two people are at one
> in their inmost hearts,
> They shatter even the strength of
> iron or of bronze.
> And when two people understand each other
> in their inmost hearts,
> Their words are sweet and strong,
> like the fragrance of orchids.[6]

Here are some suggestions that can guide you as you repair the heartmate connection.

- Share your feelings with each other.
- Let yourselves laugh and have fun.
- Cherish your time together.
- Give yourself permission to be romantic.
- Experiment with new ways to express your love.
- Make realistic plans for your future.
- Mark anniversaries of recovery.
- Celebrate being alive *and* together.

Opening Your Heart

*T*he cardiac spouse experience may seem largely a matter of coping. Six months . . . a year . . . five years down the road, you may remember this as the time you had to take care of business and try to get along the best you knew how. The countless adjustments, from medical decisions to changes in life-style, consumed your energy, attention, and time.

The cardiac crisis turned you in on yourself. Becoming more introspective and self-centered is a normal and instinctive means of self-protection. Your world got very tiny, as you concentrated on coping with your personal issues.

I remember in 1977 when a friend recommended that I read the book, Alive, a true story about the survivors of a plane crash in South America. I didn't recall ever hearing or reading about the crash in the news. When I opened the book, I was surprised to find that the date of the crash was the same day as my mother's funeral. At first I felt embarrassed about being so out of step, and wondered what else I had missed, being so absorbed in my personal pain. But when I thought about it, I could understand the natural tendency for energy to flow where it is most needed. I imagine it's the same when

*white cells rush to a wound at a specific location in the body
to provide the additional help needed for healing.*

Recovery might be defined as the gradual process of
moving back into contact with the larger world around you.
This is similar to the developmental stages children go
through as their world expands to include loyalty to and
belief in their family, their friends, then their school, their
community, state, and eventually the whole planet.

At the height of the cardiac crisis, your attention
was focused on yourself. As you emerge, you may experience dissatisfaction, restlessness, and an urge to search
your life for new meaning.

Questions about the deeper changes of your life
signal the final stop on the road to recovery. They're
different from the questions you've dealt with regarding
changes in diet and exercise, life-style, or family concerns.
They point to a new perspective, a philosophic shift, an
enhanced understanding of the meaning of life that can only
be gleaned from experience.

Before Reid's bypass surgery, everything in Susan's
life was "perfect." A self-described optimist, Susan, a forty-
six -year-old interior decorator and mother of two, always
maintained a positive attitude, no matter what problems
she confronted.

In the first few weeks following the surgery, Susan
carried on with her usual buoyancy and enthusiasm, answering all queries about Reid's health with the response,
"He's doing great, couldn't be better!"

One afternoon during Reid's nap, Susan was watching television when a public service announcement about
heart disease came on. Suddenly Susan began to cry. Without knowing why, she felt as if her heart were breaking. As
the tears flowed, Susan began to feel her disappointment,
exhaustion, and fear. She was sick and tired of pretending
that everything was fine. In that split second, she gave

herself permission to be human.

Spiritual beliefs are also tested by the cardiac crisis. Valerie, a fifty-eight-year-old cardiac spouse, struggled with doubts. Having come to her marriage with a strong religious background, she established her family's routine to include church and regular evening prayer. She taught Sunday school and was active in church activities.

After Walter's heart attack, Valerie felt that God had abandoned her. She wrestled with the question, "If there's a God, how could He allow this to happen?" She analyzed her life, trying to understand why she "deserved" such bad luck. In order to avoid feeling like a hypocrite, she turned away from the God she had trusted implicitly since childhood. She resigned from her job as Sunday school teacher, and for a while stopped attending church altogether. Questioning, as a cardiac spouse, what she had accepted blindly as a child eventually led Valerie to a renewed faith and a deeper understanding of God, herself, and her world.

The cardiac crisis is an awakening. We can no longer count on all that we once took for granted. What we didn't even notice before is now revealed to be something precious.

I wouldn't have wished heart disease on Marsh, or anyone. But it certainly woke me up. Our marriage and our lives had settled into a comfortably predictable pattern. Married for over twenty years, we had long ago lost the sense of mystery and excitement that earlier had marked our relationship. We knew each other well, had learned to sidestep our differences, and over time had softened the rough edges of our relationship. We had deepened the groove by long habit and had reached a point where we took each other for granted, not the sort of atmosphere in which growth blossoms. We had reached the "flabby forties." We were settled down and settled in.

Coming to terms with the idea of a limited *quantity* of life opens the cardiac spouse to think about *quality* of life.

As a result of your experience, you find yourself questioning your values, priorities, and beliefs. Your relationships with your mate, your family, and your spirituality are suddenly significant and genuine concerns.

We're often blind to changes within us. Beth, a thirty-year-old cardiac spouse, experienced what she described as a surprising need for spiritual support. In the middle of the night before her husband Gary's surgery, she awoke with a start. She was terrified and shaking. She tried telling herself that everything was all right and that Gary would make it through the operation. But she couldn't silence her fears. Beth got out of bed and walked outside where she stood alone in the darkness beneath the stars. Suddenly, she began to pray. Although Beth had never thought of herself as religious, her prayer was the comfort she needed at that moment. Opening her heart on that dark night was the beginning of a new faith for Beth. And her faith translated into a new career; Beth recently completed chaplaincy training and is working with cardiac families in a metropolitan hospital.

Beth's story illustrates how personal experience can translate into service—actively working to help make things better. Not everyone changes careers or makes dramatic life changes as a result of the cardiac crisis. There's only one piece of advice applicable here: Allow your heart to open, and let your open heart guide your life. Living from your heart can make your daily activity and your most important relationships a celebration of life.

Service is a natural human tendency.[1] Acting because you think you "should" or in order to "be good" is draining and exhausting. Service nourishes you as you give. We are spontaneously drawn to do service. It is the natural outpouring of the human heart.

Until I was about forty, I spent most of my energy trying to "do good" without knowing why. In retrospect, I believe that I held a deep belief that I was bad, and the only way to hide that from others and earn their love was to be a do-gooder.

I was sure that someone knew the right way to "do good" and I was determined to learn how. I experimented with various yogas, diets, meditations, and therapy. I read every self-help book I could lay my hands on. I studied various psychologies, even shifted careers, leaving teaching to become a psychotherapist, hoping that by helping others, I might get fixed too.

I was a continual disappointment to myself; my feet would fall asleep as I tried to sit in the lotus position. I felt nauseated, not enlightened by the odor of incense. I always felt either like a fraud or a failure with someone else's answers. It was like wearing the wrong pair of shoes; either they pinched because they were too tight, weren't a color that matched my clothes, or made me trip because they were so wide they fell off my feet.

One evening about a year after Marsh's bypass surgery, I accepted an invitation to a meditation service to be led by a real Tibetan lama. I arrived a few minutes late, and sat down in the back of the living room filled with chanting Americans. At first I was absorbed, not by the holiness or the mystery, but by my curiosity about how many Westerners were stuffed into one room, all shoeless, many sitting in uncomfortable poses. (At my age, the posture, if I could even get into it, would mean a sore back tomorrow for sure.) Some were chanting in a unified response to the lama, who was draped in red with a shaved head.

Once I got a sense of what was going on, I let myself wonder what I was doing there. I recalled the many evenings I had spent similarly, leaving my family and racing off to hear a speaker, an author, a teacher, a guru. And always I returned home disappointed, never finding the answer I had hoped for.

I started to think about what I had done in the past that had given me satisfaction. I recalled how meaningful it had been to create a hospital program for the families of dying patients in the early 1970s. I knew the need for the program, because of my experience at that hospital when my mother died.

My most recent work with cardiac spouses had come from my own heart as well. I felt great empathy for the unrecognized suffering and lack of support for cardiac spouses everywhere.

Sitting in that living room, while everyone chanted, I begancto understand that what is spiritual for me is participating in the human task of "making things better" when I understand the need from my own experience. I began that night to accept that I have something to offer, something to give, something that can help. I don't have to don funny clothes, assume strange postures, or eat weird foods to feel good about myself and to have a meaningful life. All I have to do is stay open, trust, and respond to the opportunities presented in my own life.

As I continue to do my work, I celebrate life by giving something back to the world. I have been richly blessed, and I have suffered. I no longer yearn to study one more discipline, or feel tempted to make the circuit for one more lecture. It's still a little scary to acknowledge that I am at peace with myself, my life, my spirituality. But each time I do, I know more surely that the way of my own heart is a spiritual way. At the same time, I feel more tolerant and compassionate toward others who are searching out their unique paths and trying to understand the meaning of their lives.

I have no intention, by sharing my own story, to push or pull any cardiac spouse toward any specific course. I have been enriched by the many cardiac spouses who have shared their lives, their struggles, and their successes with me. Some of the most beautiful stories have been the most simple. Nothing could be more stirring than heartmates expressing an increased awareness of their love, their eagerness to show it, and their courage to face the reality of their lives with increased hope for the future.

I have shared my personal story throughout this book to demonstrate that although I will always be a cardiac spouse and Marsh has heart disease forever, it didn't mean an end to all that was good in our lives. I believe that out of the cardiac experience, your life can become richer, more meaningful, and more joyous. Heart disease doesn't have to be an ending. It can be a new beginning.

APPENDIX A

Diagrams of the Heart

These four drawings illustrate the arterial blockages that cause heart attack and the bypass graft which can compensate for the damage caused by blocked arteries.

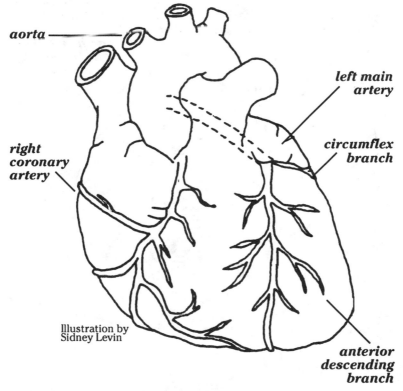

The Normal Heart

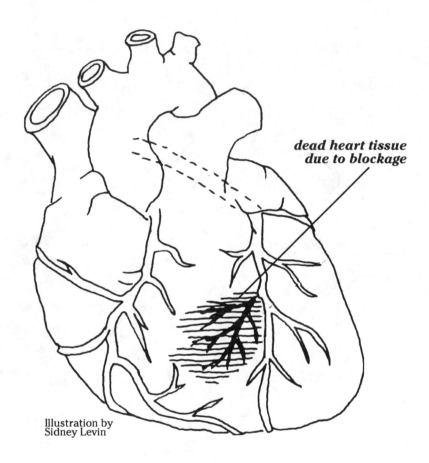

dead heart tissue
due to blockage

Illustration by
Sidney Levin

**Blockage
(Myocardial Infarction)**

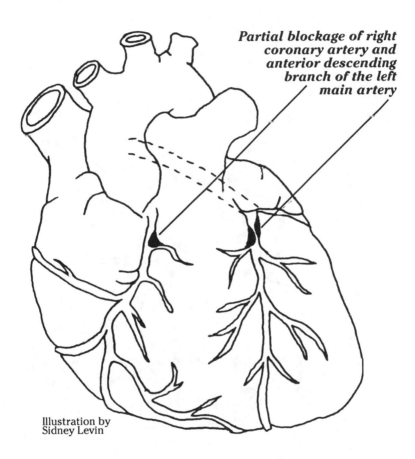

Partial blockage of right coronary artery and anterior descending branch of the left main artery

Illustration by
Sidney Levin

Partially Obstructed Heart

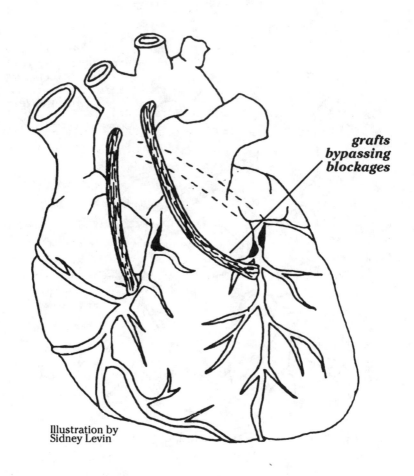

grafts
bypassing
blockages

Illustration by
Sidney Levin

Double Bypass Grafts

APPENDIX B

Self-help Tools

Relaxation

Relaxing your body and mind is a crucial component of recovery. Biofeedback and meditation are practical skills to help manage the stress of the cardiac crisis. Check local community education programs or your cardiac rehabilitation program for availability of classes.

Here is a simple exercise that requires no more than ten minutes a day. It can be done at the beginning and/or end of the day; taking ten minutes in the middle of the day can be revitalizing and energizing as well. To be effective, it should be done daily, preferably at the same time and in the same place. Have someone read the exercise to you the first few times, until you can follow the order without the distraction of having to read it.

RELAXATION EXERCISE

Sit in a comfortable chair, with your spine straight and your feet flat on the floor. Close your eyes, and focus your attention on your breath, following its natural cycle in and out. With each inhalation, be aware that you are taking in clean and clear energy. Experience the release of tension as you exhale. Allow your breathing to remain natural, don't change it in any way, just notice that with each breath you are more in touch with your depth and you become more relaxed.

Focus now on your body so that it can relax and you can let go of the tension you carry there. Begin with your feet: first your right foot, then your left. Imagine all of the tension flowing out through the bottom of your feet and into the earth below. Now allow the muscles in your calves and thighs to relax as well. First your right leg, then, your left. Your legs feel warm and loose. Now pay attention to your abdomen, where you may feel tightness and stress. Let your breath flow through your abdomen, and let go of the tension. Now focus on your back with its many muscles, and your shoulders. Breathe energy into your shoulders, and feel the tension let go. Now attend to your arms, first the right, then, the left. Let go, first in your upper arm, then the lower part, and last your hands. Experience the tightness flowing out of every fingertip. Feel your neck relaxed and free as the tension flows from it. Concentrate now on your jaw, letting it relax, letting your mouth open naturally as you let go of holding it tight. Now focus on your eyes and allow them to let go. Feel the muscles behind your eyes relaxing and expanding. And last, the top and back of your head. Feel your head get light and clear as your mind stops racing. You are alert but not busy. Now that your body is relaxed, focus once again on your breath. Breathe in whatever quality you need at this moment—calm, peace, serenity, freedom, love—and exhale any remaining tension or tightness.

Imagine yourself in a beautiful green meadow. You are able to rest and be nurtured by the beauty of nature surrounding you. You feel the warm sun on your skin, the solid earth holds you securely. The air is fresh and there is a pleasant cool breeze. You can smell grasses and wildflowers. You hear birds singing and the babble of a nearby brook. Take some time to enjoy the peace and the calm. Allow yourself to be filled and quieted.

Stay in this serene and beautiful place as long as you are comfortable. When you are ready, focus your attention on your breath again. Breathe as fully and deeply as you naturally can. Notice how you feel as you do. Now, very gently, bring your awareness back to the present and slowly open your eyes. Take a moment to stretch your body as tall as you can when you rise and return to your everyday reality.

The Evening Review

The Evening Review is a daily exercise designed to enhance personal growth. It is particularly useful to the cardiac spouse because it provides a structure to establish regular introspection, a quiet time when you can think about your day. It can help you to focus on questions about life raised by the cardiac crisis. The process of doing the exercise facilitates acceptance of reality, in regular and small steps.

The Evening Review can be used as a recovery tool, helping the cardiac spouse to focus on him- or herself. Reviewing is a mental activity, naturally operating during a crisis, that helps a person to think clearly, see reality, and establish order in the chaos of the crisis.

EVENING REVIEW EXERCISE

The review is best done as the last activity of your day. Before going to sleep, review your day in your mind, "playing" it like a movie, backward, beginning where you are right now, then the time of late evening, then the time of early evening, then the dinner hour, the afternoon, and so on to the morning when you awakened.

This exercise can be used to examine yourself and your life as a whole. It can be modified, as in the example below, to focus on some aspect of yourself, on some inner process or pattern you'd like to know more about. The attitude with which you do the exercise is most important. When you examine your day, do it as much as possible as the detached "objective observer," calmly and clearly registering each phase of what has happened. Then move on to the next phase without excitement, without becoming elated at a success or unhappy about a failure. The aim is to calmly register awareness of the meaning and patterns of the day, rather than relive it.

Many have found it valuable to write down, perhaps as part of a journal or your Heartmates® diary, observations, insights, or impressions. By reviewing your notes over a period of time, you may discover patterns and trends not otherwise apparent.

REVIEW OF BOUNDARIES

This modification of the Evening Review consists of reviewing your day from the point of view of your boundaries. Psychological boundaries are protective membranes best used to deflect what is detrimental to the system and to attract what nourishes it. (Consider how skillfully a plant protects itself from poisonous or unneeded elements and finds nutrients in the appropriate quantities to sustain its growth.)

Before doing this exercise the first time, you might identify activities and relationships that are particularly nourishing or depleting at this point in your life. If you keep a journal, reviewing recent writings may provide insight.

As part of your Evening Review, some of the things you may want to keep in mind are:[1]

1. What is my experience of my boundaries? Have there been changes in my boundary system since the cardiac crisis began? Are there changes as I become aware of my boundaries and how I use them?

2. How do I evaluate environmental influences? From which can I get nourishment or from which do I need protection?

3. How skillful am I in using and shifting my boundaries? In what situations and with whom is it easy or difficult?

4. What do I allow In? What do I push away? What in myself do I protect (my heart, my mind, my body, my feelings)?

You may consider these questions during the review exercise itself, or, if this gets in your way, you may want to think about them at the end of your review. They are meant to provide a choice of perspective and all need not be covered. Their main purpose is to increase awareness of your boundaries and protection.

Keep the exercise simple, and particularly at the beginning give it no more than fifteen minutes a day (including journal writing).

Partial Life Review

In the confusion of loss, it is the search for meaning that brings people from dark times into the light. One of the natural ways people search is by reviewing what has happened to them in a crisis. This exercise is designed to assist cardiac spouses by structuring a way to look at a transition or loss in their past, before the cardiac crisis.

The exercise is particularly useful to find qualities and strengths already developed that have application in the present crisis. Looking at how you handled a loss or crisis in the past can familiarize you with your patterns of coping. It's likely that you will find similarities in your coping skills now. Looking at your patterns is the first step to incorporating the best of what you have done with new choices.

You may want to do the exercise more than once, focusing on other transitions you have experienced. When you are familiar with the process, you can use the exercise to look at the cardiac crisis you are experiencing in the present. Keep writing materials near; insights (like dreams) are quickly forgotten unless they are written down.

PARTIAL LIFE REVIEW EXERCISE[2]

Take a few minutes to reflect on several periods of transition or events that were turning points in your life. Begin by jotting them down on paper. They might include a major decision you made some time ago, the loss of a relationship that has affected you, or something that happened on a larger scale, outside yourself, that has had an influence on your life.

Now, from those events you have written down choose one that you are willing to look at in a more detailed way.

First, recall the period of your life when the event happened. What was going on within you, outside you? Who were the important people in your life? Was there a person or persons that you confided in? Were you alone, without support? As you review this period of your life, see yourself as you were then.

Now recall how you acted, what kinds of things you did at the time of the event (the decision, transition, choice, loss). What was your behavioral response to the event itself?

As you see yourself in retrospect, how did you feel about what was happening to you? Notice the progression of feelings that occurred as the experience happened. Your feelings at the onset of the period may have been very different from what you felt later as you integrated the experience into your life. Notice, too, whether you expressed your feelings directly then, or whether you pushed them down or away. Did you express some feelings and suppress others? As you look back, can you see any of your feelings being expressed indirectly? Did anyone important to you know how you were feeling then?

Shift your focus of attention to your thoughts at the time of the event. What were you aware of, considering, weighing, judging? Notice whether you did that thinking alone or whether there was someone you discussed those thoughts with. At that time did you think that what was happening was an opportunity? Did it make sense to you in the larger context of your life?

Now, bring yourself and your awareness back to the present, being aware that whatever the event was, you are beyond it now. With the passage of time, and reviewing it now, does the event make sense in relation to your life? Is there something you can see about it now that you couldn't see then? Does reviewing this particular event change how you see yourself, your image? Are you now more understanding, judgmental, compassionate, accepting, forgiving of what you did, how you felt, or what you thought of yourself then? Is there anything you learned then (a skill or a quality that was developed) that can be useful to you in your life now?

Is there anything in this review that points toward your future . . . any new way you'd like to act or live, think, or feel, having looked clearly at the past? What are the implications for the future, now that you have reviewed the past in this way?

When you have finished looking, take time to write about what you've learned. If it makes sense to continue the process, you may want to share your review with someone important in your life. You may want to focus on this event, its implications, and the pattern(s) revealed in a regular Evening Review for a period of time.

Family Meeting: Problem-solving Model

When difficult decisions need to be made and long-term changes need to be accepted and integrated, families may feel vulnerable and unprepared. Old conflicts may erupt to complicate the present issues. New roles and evolving family rules may need to be clarified. Establishing regular family council meetings to discuss problems and seek solutions is one way to deal with the cardiac crisis as a family.

Family council meetings should be scheduled for a definite day and time, weekly. Each meeting should be led by a different member of the family. The responsibility of record-keeping (in summary or "minutes" form) should also be shared. Meetings should be no longer than one hour. Family members of all ages should be included, if possible. I recommend that children as young as elementary school age attend. They will learn from being included, even if they have little to contribute at first.

The family will experience success if all members are willing to approach issues as *family* problems. The solution to problems is as much a family responsibility as are the problems. This approach develops mutual respect and cooperation and promotes family support and cohesion.

Here is a six-step guide your family can follow to solve problems together.

1. Together make a list of all the family concerns. Anything unresolved in the eyes of one family member belongs on the list. Be wary of commenting on contributions. This is not the place or the time to share feelings about any one problem. Don't permit anyone to blame anyone else for any problem. The purpose of this family activity is to seek solutions to the dilemmas of the family.

2. Together, select the three to five most critical issues. Selection should take into account which issues are the most pressing and which are the most important. The remainder of the list should be deferred for discussion at a later time.

3. Together, define what information is needed and which family members are responsible for data collection. The goal of this step in the problem-solving process is to gather all the ideas, information, and outside resources that will help the family to resolve the issues. Individual family members should also reflect on their own ideas about each of the critical problems during this period of time.

4. Meet together to share information and resources. The purpose of this meeting is to share all the information and ideas on each of the critical issues to be resolved. Respect for each person's ideas and attentive listening to the data gathered are essential for success at this step.

5. Share individual ideas for solutions/resolutions. Every solution offered by family members should be heard and considered. One family member can be designated as secretary for each issue, responsible to put each solution in writing. The most pressing problem should be discussed first, followed by the others in the priority of their importance.

6. Together, agree on a best solution. By consensus, negotiation, and compromise, the family agrees to a resolution. The family also needs to decide what actions will accomplish resolution, and what each family member needs to do. Before a next set of issues is taken on by the family, there should be a follow-up meeting to assure that resolution on issues being worked on is complete. Celebrate each solution as a family!

APPENDIX C

Heartmates® Recommended Reading List

Borysenko, Joan, *Fire In The Soul: A New Psychology of Spiritual Optimism.* New York: Warner Books, 1993.

Bozarth-Campbell, Alla, *Life is Good-bye, Life is Hello: Grieving Well Through All Kinds of Loss.* Minneapolis, Minn.: Compcare Publications, 1982.

Brecher, Edward, *Love, Sex and Aging.* Boston: Little, Brown & Co., 1984.

Bridges, William, *Transitions, Making Sense of Life's Changes,* Reading, Mass.: Addison-Wesley Publishing Co., 1980.

Colgrove, Melba, Ph.D., Harold H. Bloomfield, M.D., and Peter McWilliams, *How to Survive the Loss of a Love, 58 Things to Do When There is Nothing to Be Done.* New York: Bantam Books, 1977.

Cousins, Norman, *The Healing Heart.* New York: W.W. Norton & Co., 1983.

Doerr, Harriet, *Stones for Ibarra.* New York: Penguin Books, 1978.

Ericsson, Stephanie, *Companion Through the Darkness: Inner Dialogues on Grief.* New York: HarperCollins, 1993.

Halperin, Jonathan L., M.D., and Richard Levine, *Bypass.* New York: Random House, 1985.

Hazelton, Lesley, *The Right to Feel Bad.* New York: Random House, 1984.

Hoffman, Nancy Yanes, *Change of Heart: The Bypass Experience.* New York: Harcourt Brace Jovanovich, 1985.

Kenney, Susan, *Sailing.* New York: Viking Penguin Inc., 1988.

Kushner, Harold S., *When Bad Things Happen to Good People.* New York: Schocken Books, Inc., 1981.

L'Engle, Madeleine, *Two-Part Invention, The Story of A Marriage.* New York: Farrar, Straus & Giroux, 1988.

Lerner, Harriet Goldhor, Ph.D., *The Dance of Anger: A Woman's Guide to Changing the Patterns of Intimate Relationships.* New York: Harper & Row, 1986.

Lerner, Harriet Goldhor, Ph.D., *The Dance of Intimacy: A Woman's Guide to Courageous Acts of Change in Key Relationships.* New York: Harper & Row, 1989.

Scarf, Maggie, *Intimate Partners: Patterns in Love and Marriage.* New York: Random House, 1987.

Scheingold, L.D., and N. Wagner, *Sound Sex and the Aging Heart.* New York: Human Sciences Press, 1974.

Schover, Leslie, *Prime Time: Sexual Health for Men over Fifty.* New York: Holt, Rinehart & Winston, 1984.

Siegel, Bernie S., M.D., *Love, Medicine & Miracles.* New York: Harper & Row, 1986.

Sotile, Wayne M., Ph.D., *Heart Illness and Intimacy, How Caring Relationships Aid Recovery.* Baltimore: The Johns Hopkins University Press, 1992.

Strong, Maggie, *Mainstay: For the Well Spouse of the Chronically Ill.* Boston: Little, Brown & Co., 1988.

Tatelbaum, Judy, *The Courage to Grieve.* New York: Perennial Library, Harper & Row, 1980.

Veninga, Robert, *A Gift of Hope.* Boston: Little, Brown & Co., 1985.

Viorst, Judith, *Necessary Losses.* New York: Simon & Schuster, 1986.

Chapter Notes

CHAPTER 1
1. Refer to appendix A for diagrams of healthy, damaged, and bypassed hearts. See glossary for clarification of medical terminology.

CHAPTER 2
1. My favorite cardiac cookbook is *Craig Claiborne's Gourmet Diet*, written by Craig Claiborne with Pierre Franey. (New York: Ballantine Books, 1980). It includes low-sodium and modified-cholesterol recipes. Our favorite recipe is the Lemon Chicken, Texas style.

CHAPTER 3
1. See Stephanie Ericsson's *Companion Through The Darkness: Inner Dialogues on Grief,* (New York: HarperCollins, 1993), for an eloquent and elegant experience of grieving. About anger, she says it is "...our natural protective armor. It tells the rest of the world that a boundary has been violated. Our society would have us swallow it, and many of us do....Rage is white-hot anger....It is a superb emotion. Used correctly, it lays down permanent boundaries, stakes out lifetime territories, and gives us girth. It will launch us out of inertia and thrust us forward." page 67.
2. Lesley Hazelton, *The Right to Feel Bad* (New York: Ballantine Books, 1984), pp. 196-197.
3. Henry David Thoreau, *Walden* (New York: Modern Library, 1950), p. 290.
4. It is useful to differentiate between needless guilt and guilt that is healthy and appropriate. See Judith Viorst, "Good as Guilt," chapter 9 in her book *Necessary Losses* (New York: Fawcett Gold Medal, 1986), pp. 150-151, for a discussion of the healing value of making reparations for the wrongful act done.
5. Heartmates® Feelings and Needs Assessment Diary is adapted from Ellen Sue Stern, *Expecting Change* (New York: Poseidon Press, 1986), pp. 114-115.

225

CHAPTER 4
1. Rhoda F. Levin, : "Life Review: A Natural Process," in *Readings in Psychosynthesis: Theory, Process, and Practice* (Toronto, Canada: OISE), pp. 82-96.

CHAPTER 5
1. Stanton Peele and Archie Brodsky, *Love and Addiction* (New York: New American Library, 1975), p. 6.
2. Robert Eliot, M.D., *Stress and the Major Cardiovascular Disorders* (Mt. Kisco, N.Y.: Futura Publishing Co., 1979), p. 14.
3. Hans Selye, M.D., *The Stress of Life* (New York: McGraw Hill Book Co., 1956), p. 299.

CHAPTER 6
1. Jean Shinoda Bolen, M.D., *The Tao of Psychology, Synchronicity, and the Self* (San Francisco: Harper & Row, 1979), p. 2.

CHAPTER 7
1. Hippocrates, Precepts, chapter 1, Quoted in John Bartlett, *Familiar Quotations*, 13th ed. (Boston: Little, Brown & Co., 1955), p. 21.
2. Elizabeth Kübler-Ross, *On Death and Dying* (New York: Macmillan, 1969).
3. Amelia Earhart Putnam, *Courage* Quoted in John Bartlett, *Familiar Quotations*, 13th ed. (Boston: Little, Brown & Co., 1955), p. 981.
4. William Shakespeare, Macbeth, Act IV, Scene iii, in *Twenty-three Plays and Sonnets*, ed. Thomas Marc Parrott (New York: Charles Scribner's Sons, 1953), p. 853.
5. F. Scott Fitzgerald, *The Great Gatsby* (New York: Charles Scribner's Sons, 1953), p. 105.
6. Carl Simonton, S. Simonton, and J. Creighton, *Getting Well Again* (Los Angeles: Tarcher, 1978); and Jeanne Achterberg, *Imagery in Healing* (Boston: New Science Library, 1985).
7. Adapted from a broadcast on Minnesota Public Radio entitled "Positive Emotions and Health," on 8/9/85. Presented by Norman Cousins at St. John's Hospital and Medical Center, Santa Monica, California.

CHAPTER 8
1. Edward J. Speedling, *Heart Attack: The Family Response at Home and in the Hospital* (New York: Tavistock Publications, 1982), p. 162.
2. Theodore Isaac Rubin, M.D., *The Angry Book* (New York: Macmillan, 1969), pp. 168-169.
3. Thomas Hackett, M.D., *"Men and Sex after a Heart Attack,"* Harvard Medical School Health Letter, Vol. 11, No. 5 (March, 1986), pp. 5-6.
4. Ibid., p. 6.
5. Ibid., p. 6.
6. Quoted from the I Ching. In Ram Dass and Paul Gorman, *How Can I Help?* (New York: Alfred A. Knopf, 1985), p. 114.

CHAPTER 9
1. See the section on "Service" in John Firman's and James Vargiu's article "Dimensions of Growth," in *Synthesis 3-4*, available only in libraries. Also see Ram Dass and Paul Gorman's book, *How Can I Help?* (New York: Alfred A. Knopf, 1985), an elegant and touching study of the simplicity of service.

APPENDIX B
1. Adapted from the unpublished writings of Roberto Assagioli.
2. Adapted from Rhoda F. Levin, "Life Review: A Natural Process," in *Readings in Psychosynthesis: Theory, Process, and Practice* (Toronto: Ontario Institute for Studies in Education, 1985), p. 96.

GLOSSARY
Medical Terms

Angina. The heart muscle's complaint that it is not receiving enough blood or oxygen. It frequently occurs when the heart works harder than usual, such as during exercise, stress, sexual intercourse, walking in extremely hot or cold weather, or after eating a large meal. Anginal discomfort can be experienced in a variety of ways. It can feel like chest pain, pressure, or heaviness. It can feel like a pain or ache in the jaw, teeth, or earlobes, or be a choking or tightening sensation in the throat. It can be experienced as pain, aching, or numbness in one or both arms or hands, between the shoulder blades, or in the neck. Anginal discomfort may start in one place and move to another (i.e. chest pain that spreads to the shoulder and down the arm). It is important to know that angina is not just felt as "chest pain," but as a variety of symptoms. Angina is usually brief (from thirty seconds to five minutes) and may disappear slowly or quickly. Angina is not a heart attack.

Aneurysm. A weakness in an artery or vein in the wall of your heart muscle that forms a balloonlike bulge.

Angiogram. An X-ray picture of the coronary arteries. In the procedure, a catheter (specialized tube) is inserted into an artery in the groin. It follows the artery's path up to the heart, where, through the tube, dye is injected while filming is done. These films show areas of narrowing or blockage in the coronary arteries and help the cardiologist and cardiac surgeon plan the most effective treatment. This procedure takes about an hour and has some risk involved, but it is the most precise reading of coronary artery blockage available. After the procedure, the patient must lie flat for a number of hours to prevent the artery from reopening and bleeding.

Aorta. The large main artery that leaves the heart delivering freshly oxygenated blood to all parts of the body.

Arrhythmia. Any change in the normal rhythm of the heart.

Arteries. These are the blood vessels that carry fresh (oxygenated) blood from the heart to all parts of the body. (Veins are the blood vessels that bring used blood back to the heart.)

Arteriosclerosis. A progressive condition that causes the artery walls to thicken and lose their elasticity. Also called "hardening of the arteries."

Atherosclerosis. This is a form of arteriosclerosis, in which the passageways through the arteries become roughened and narrowed by fatty deposits (see "Plaque") that harden along the inner lining of the arteries.

Balloon angioplasty. A procedure used to open clogged arteries. A special balloon catheter (tube) is inserted into an artery in the groin, as in the angiogram procedure. The catheter is positioned into the narrowed portion of the coronary artery, and the balloon is inflated. The balloon compresses the plaque, widening the narrowed area of the passageway, to increase the flow of blood and oxygen to the heart muscle.

Bypass surgery. (also referred to as coronary artery bypass surgery, CAB, CABS) This operation uses a blood vessel from another part of the body to bypass the blocked area in the coronary artery (see diagram). A clean blood vessel is sewn above and below the blockage in the coronary artery. It is the construction of a new pathway for blood to flow around the narrowed section of artery to the heart muscle. Picture the surgery as providing a detour around a traffic jam, so that cars can get where they're going unimpeded. The procedure should improve the blood flow to the heart muscle. Angina is relieved for 90 percent of those who have bypass surgery.

Blood enzyme test. Cardiac enzymes are substances that are normally stored in the heart muscle. During an injury to the heart (i.e. a heart attack), these enzymes are released into the blood stream. Several blood samples are drawn after a suspected heart attack to check for these enzymes. This blood test helps to determine whether or not a heart attack has occurred. It usually takes twenty-four to forty-eight hours after the suspected heart attack to get results.

Blood Pressure. The pressure placed on the walls of your arteries as your heart pumps blood. The top number (systolic) refers to the pressure in your arteries while your heart is contracting, and the bottom number (diastolic) refers to the pressure in your arteries when your heart is relaxed (in between beats). Hypertension is high blood pressure, usually greater than 140 over 90 in adults.

Cardiac risk factors. These are living habits, physical attributes, and characteristics or inherited tendencies that may increase the chance of developing heart disease. Risk factors include: smoking, high blood pressure, high blood cholesterol, inactivity, obesity, diabetes, stress, and heredity.

Cholesterol. A fat-like substance found only in animal products (highest in organ meats), dairy products, and eggs. The cholesterol present in our blood stream originates from the cholesterol we eat plus what we produce ourselves. Elevated blood cholesterol is associated with an increased risk of atherosclerosis. Cholesterol can be broken down (see "Lipoproteins").

Congestive heart failure. A condition in which a weakened heart is not able to adequately pump the blood around the body. Poor circulation results, and fluid may collect in the lungs, ankles, and feet.

Coronary arteries. Three main arteries and their branches (see diagram), that supply the heart muscle with blood, oxygen, and nutrients. If these arteries become narrowed by atherosclerosis, angina or a heart attack can occur.

CPR (Cardiopulmonary resuscitation). A lifesaving skill, often called mouth-to-mouth resuscitation, that is taught by the American Red Cross. I recommend that all cardiac spouses become certified in CPR. Preparation and training my help you save a life. You will also gain confidence in your ability to respond appropriately and efficiently in an emergency.

Echocardiogram. A way of viewing the heart without entering the body. This technique uses high frequency sound waves for measuring and determining the function and structure of the heart. It is completely painless and takes from one half to one hour to complete. Echocardiograms cannot see coronary arteries at this time, and therefore cannot be used to pinpoint the narrowed arteries (see "Angiogram").

EKG (Electrocardiogram). A recording of the electrical currents produced by the heart. These electrical currents are responsible for the beating of the heart muscle. A resting EKG can detect any abnormal beats and can determine if the heart muscle is presently not receiving enough blood and oxygen, or if heart damage was done in the past. It is a painless procedure of attaching suction cups to the skin.

Endotracheal tube. A tube placed in the windpipe through which air and oxygen are passed to aid breathing, used in surgery or with very ill patients. Bypass patients complain about the frustration of this tube because they can't speak. Having a pad and pencil, small chalkboard, or "magic slate" available can enhance the patient's ability to communicate until the tube is removed (usually twenty-four to forty-eight hours after surgery).

Exercise. Forms of physical activity done by cardiac patients for the purposes of reducing risk factors, increasing physical fitness, and possibly improving cardiac function and the quality of life. The activities that seem to produce these results are walking, jogging, bicycling, swimming, and rowing (aerobic exercises). It is generally recommended that individuals with heart disease engage in these activities three to five times a week for a twenty- to forty-five minute session. Check with your personal physician for more specific guidelines.

Heart Attack. (Also called a myocardial infarction, an "MI," or a coronary thrombosis.) This occurs when the flow of blood to a part of the heart muscle is suddenly cut off or severely diminished. A part of the heart muscle dies in a heart attack. (See diagram.)

Lipoproteins (HDL, LDL). Fats carried in the blood, also known as "good cholesterol" (HDL) and "bad cholesterol" (LDL). Abnormal levels of these fats are associated with heart and blood vessel disease. Triglycerides are another type of fat found in the bloodstream; a modest elevation of triglycerides is probably not an important risk factor for heart disease, unless the blood cholesterol is also elevated. High triglyceride levels are found more commonly in overweight and/or diabetic individuals, who consume a high fat diet.

MEDICATIONS:

Anticoagulants. (Also referred to incorrectly as "blood thinners," they do not actually thin the blood). These medications are used to improve the flow of blood and prevent the formation of blood clots. (Blood clots blocking the coronary arteries can cause a heart attack.)

Antiarrhythmics. These are a group of medications that regulate irregular heart rhythms.

Antihypertensives. Medications of many types, used to lower high blood pressure.

Betablockers. A group of medications used to treat high blood pressure. Some beta blockers are used to help relieve angina, and are taken to help prevent additional heart attacks. One side effect of betablockers is reduced libido or impotency.

Often switching to a different betablocker will eliminate the side effect.

Calcium channel blockers. A group of medications used to treat angina by increasing the supply of blood and oxygen to the heart while reducing the work of the heart.

Cholesterol reducers. Medication that lowers the level of cholesterol in the blood.

Diuretics. Medications that increase the output of urine, there fore helping to reduce the amount of fluid and sodium in the body. They can be used to treat high blood pressure and congestive heart failure.

Nitrates. Medication commonly prescribed to treat angina. They work by increasing the supply of blood and oxygen to the heart, while reducing the work of the heart. They may be prescribed in several forms: a tablet to be dissolved under the tongue, a tablet to be swallowed, an ointment or a patch to be applied to the skin.

Nitroglycerin. A commonly prescribed fast-acting medication used to treat angina (see "nitrates").

Vasodilators. A group of medications that dilate blood vessels, which increases the blood flow to that area.

Pacemaker. A mechanical implant that stimulates and regulates the heartbeat by a series of regular electrical discharges.

Plaque. In heart disease, this refers to a patchy deposit of fatty material consisting of cholesterol, calcium, and other materials, found on the inner lining of the coronary arteries.

Post cardiotomy syndrome. (or "post myocardial infarction syndrome" or "Dressler's syndrome"). A condition of inflammation in the sack covering the heart, occurring after a heart attack or heart surgery. It is characterized by fever and chest pain (different than angina or incision pain). It is treatable with anti-inflammatory medications such as aspirin or cortisone.

Saturated fat. A type of fat usually solid at room temperature. Common sources include animal products (butter, chicken skin, marbled meats), and some vegetable products (coconut oil, palm oil, cocoa butter, and hydrogenated vegetable oils). High dietary intake of saturated fat tends to elevate the level of cholesterol in the blood. Limiting foods high in saturated fats helps to lower blood cholesterol. The U.S. Senate's Select Committee on Nutrition and Human Needs suggests reducing the intake of dietary fat to 30 percent of diet, and reducing cholesterol intake to 300 milligrams daily.

Sodium. A mineral, most commonly found in table salt. Sodium retains fluid in the body, which can increase the work of the heart and increase blood pressure. It is usually recommended that individuals with high blood pressure or heart disease restrict the amount of sodium in their diets. There are high levels of sodium in prepared and frozen foods. Two thousand milligrams daily is a sensible level to try to maintain.

Streptokinase. An enzyme (or substance) that can dissolve blood clots. If given immediately after a heart attack begins, it can help prevent heart muscle damage. (Atenolol, a drug being used experimentally in 1986, if injected soon after a heart attack begins and is taken orally for a week, can ease the heart's workload and reduce the risk of having another heart attack, or a cardiac arrest.)

Stress Test. (Also called a "graded exercise test," or a "GXT"). This procedure tests how well the heart delivers oxygenated blood during physical exertion. It is done for several purposes: It can help determine the level of fitness, be used for prescribing safe exercise levels, and/or determine the presence of heart disease. There is no such thing as passing or failing the stress test. With a doctor present, the person having a stress test is attached to an EKG machine and begins walking on a treadmill. The treadmill is started at a slow speed and elevation, and both are gradually increased. Blood pressure and EKG are monitored closely for changes in blood pressure and/or heartbeats.

Unsaturated fat. Includes polyunsaturated and monounsaturated fats, both of which help to lower the level of cholesterol in the blood. Major sources of polyunsaturated fat include liquid vegetable oils such as corn, sunflower, cottonseed, safflower and soybean oil. Polyunsaturated fats tend to lower blood cholesterol. Monounsaturated fats are found in peanuts, peanut oil, olives, and olive oil. The general recommendation is to limit total fat intake to 30 percent of the total calories, one-third from each of the three types of fat: polyunsaturated, monounsaturated, and saturated fat.

BIBLIOGRAPHY

Achterberg, Jeanne. *Imagery in Healing.* Boston: New Science Library, 1985.

Alexander, Jo, Debi Berrow, Lisa Domitrovich, Margarita Donnelly, and Cheryl McLean, eds. *Women and Aging.* Corvalis, Ore.: Calyx Books, 1986.

Assagioli, Roberto. *The Act of Will.* New York: Viking Press, 1973.

_____. *Psychosynthesis: A Manual of Principles and Techniques.* New York: Penguin Books, 1965.

Bolen, Jean Shinoda, M.D. *Goddesses in Every Woman.* New York: Harper & Row, 1984.

_____. *The Tao of Psychology, Synchronicity and the Self.* San Francisco: Harper & Row, 1979.

Boston Women's Health Book Collective. *Our Bodies, Ourselves.* New York: Simon & Schuster, 1971.

Bozarth-Campbell, Alla. *Life is Good-bye, Life is Hello: Grieving Well Through All Kinds of Loss.* Minneapolis: Compcare Publications, 1982.

Brecher, Edward. *Love, Sex and Aging.* Boston: Little, Brown & Co., 1984.

Bridges, William. *Transitions, Making Sense of Life's Changes.* Reading, Mass.: Addison-Wesley Publishing Co., 1980.

Budnick, Herbert N., Ph.D. with Scott Robert Hays. *Heart to Heart, A Guide to the Psychological Aspects of Heart Disease.* Santa Fe: HealthPress, 1991.

Colgrove, Melba, Ph.D., Harold H. Bloomfield, M.D., and Peter McWilliams. *How to Survive the Loss of a Love.* New York: Bantam Books, 1977.

Cousins, Norman. *Anatomy of an Illness.* New York: W.W. Norton & Co., Inc., 1979.

_____. *The Healing Heart.* New York: W.W. Norton & Co., 1983.

Craven, Margaret. *I Heard the Owl Call My Name.* Garden City, N.Y.: Doubleday, 1973.

Davidson, Glen W. *Understanding Mourning: A Guide for Those Who Grieve.* Minneapolis: Augsburg Press, 1984.

235

Doerr, Harriet. *Stones for Ibarra.* New York: Penguin Books, 1978.

Doress, Paula Brown, Diana Laskin Siegal & The Midlife and Older Women Book Project. *Ourselves, Growing Older.* New York: Simon & Schuster, 1987.

Dreikurs, Rudolf, M.D., and Vicki Soltz. *Children: The Challenge.* New York: Hawthorn Books, 1964.

Eliot, Robert, M.D. *Stress and the Major Cardiovascular Disorders.* Mt. Kisco, N.Y.: Futura Publishing Co., 1979.

Ericsson, Stephanie, *Companion Through the Darkness: Inner Dialogues on Grief.* New York: HarperCollins, 1993.

Ferrucci, Piero. *Inevitable Grace.* Los Angeles: J.P. Tarcher, 1990.

_____. *What We May Be.* Los Angeles: J.P. Tarcher, 1982.

Firman, John, and James Vargiu. "Dimensions of Growth," in *Synthesis 3-4.* Redwood City, Calif.: Synthesis Press, 1977.

Fossum, Merle A. and Marilyn J. Mason. *Facing Shame: Families in Recovery.* New York: W.W. Norton & Co., 1986.

Fowler, James W. *Stages of Faith.* San Francisco: Harper & Row, 1981.

Friedman, Meyer, M.D., and Ray H. Rosenman, M.D. *Type A Behavior and Your Heart.* New York: Fawcett Publications, 1974.

Gilligan, Carol. *In a Different Voice.* Cambridge, Mass.: Harvard University Press, 1982.

Halperin, Jonathan L., M.D., and Richard Levine. *Bypass.* New York: Times Books, 1985.

Hazleton, Lesley. *The Right to Feel Bad.* New York: Ballantine Books, 1984.

Hoffman, Nancy Yanes. *Change of Heart: The Bypass Experience.* New York: Harcourt Brace Jovanovich, 1985.

Jung, Carl. *Memories, Dreams, Reflections.* New York: Vintage Books, 1965.

Kavanaugh, Robert E. *Facing Death.* Baltimore: Penguin Books, 1972.

Kegan, Robert. *The Evolving Self.* Cambridge, Mass.: Harvard University Press, 1982.

Kenney, Susan. *Sailing.* New York: Viking Penguin Inc., 1988.

Klagsbrun, Francine. *Married People: Staying Together in the Age of Divorce.* New York: Bantam Books, 1985.

Kopp, Sheldon. *Raise Your Right Hand Against Fear, Extend the Other in Compassion.* New York: Ballantine Books, 1988.

Kübler-Ross, Elizabeth, M.D. *On Death and Dying.* New York: Macmillan Co., 1969.

Kushner, Harold S. *When All You've Ever Wanted Isn't Enough: The Search for a Life That Matters.* New York: Simon & Schuster, 1986.

_____. *When Bad Things Happen To Good People.* New York: Schocken Books, 1981.

Larsen, Earnie. *Stage II Recovery: Life Beyond Addiction.* Minneapolis: Winston Press, 1965.

Laurence, Margaret. *The Stone Angel.* Toronto: McClelland & Stewart, 1964.

Lear, Martha Weinman. *Heartsounds.* New York: Simon & Schuster, 1980.

L'Engle, Madeleine. *Two-Part Invention, The Story of A Marriage.* New York: Farrar, Straus & Giroux, 1988.

Leonard, Linda Scheirse. *The Wounded Woman.* Boulder, Colo.: Shambhala, 1983.

Lerner, Harriet Goldhor, Ph.D. *The Dance of Anger: A Woman's Guide to Changing the Patterns of Intimate Relationships.* New York: Harper & Row, 1986.

_____. The *Dance of Intimacy: A Woman's Guide to Courageous Acts of Change in Key Relationships.* New York: Harper & Row, 1989.

Lessing, Doris. *The Summer Before the Dark.* New York: Vintage Books, 1973.

Levin, Rhoda F. "Life Review: A Natural Process," in *Readings in Psychosynthesis: Theory, Process, and Practice.* Toronto: OISE, 1985.

Lewis, C.S. *A Grief Observed.* New York: Bantam Books, 1961.

_____. *The Four Loves.* New York: Harcourt, Brace, Jovanovich, 1960.

Lifton, Robert J, and Eric Olson. *Living and Dying.* New York. New York: Bantam Books, 1984.

Lindemann, Erich, M.D. *Beyond Grief: Studies in Crisis Intervention.* New York: Jason Aronson, Inc., 1979.

Lynch, James J. *The Broken Heart: The Medical Consequences of Loneliness.* New York: Basic Books, 1977.

Maslow, Abraham H. *The Farther Reaches of Human Nature.* New York: Penguin Books, 1971.

Miller, Alice. *Thou Shalt Not Be Aware.* New York: New American Library, 1984.

Moustakas, Clark E. *Loneliness and Love.* Englewood Cliffs, N.J.: Prentice-Hall, Inc., 1972.

Napier, Augustus Y., Ph.D., and Carl A. Whitaker, M.D. *The Family*

Crucible. New York: Bantam Books, 1978.

Needleman, Jacob. *The Heart of Philosophy.* New York: Bantam Books, 1982.

_____. *A Sense of the Cosmos.* New York: E.P. Dutton & CO., 1975.

Ornish, Dean, M.D. *Eat More, Weigh Less.* New York: HarperCollins, 1993.

_____. *Program for Reversing Heart Disease.* New York: Random House, 1990.

_____. *Stress, Diet, & Your Heart.* New York: Holt, Rinehart & Winston, 1982.

Peck, M. Scott, M.D. *The Road Less Traveled.* New York: Simon & Schuster, 1978.

Peele, Stanton. *Love and Addiction.* New York: New American Library, 1975.

Pincus, Lily. *Death and the Family.* New York: Random House, 1974.

Ram Dass and Paul Gorman. *How Can I Help?* New York: Alfred A. Knopf, 1985.

Rogers, Natalie. *Emerging Woman: A Decade of Midlife Transitions.* Point Reyes, Calif.: Personal Press, 1980.

Rubin, Lillian. *Intimate Strangers: Men and Women Together.* New York: Harper & Row, 1983.

_____. *Women of a Certain Age.* New York: Harper & Row, 1979.

Rubin, Theodore Isaac, M.D. *The Angry Book.* New York: Macmillan Co., 1969.

Sarton, May. *Kinds of Love.* New York: W.W. Norton & Co., 1970.

Scarf, Maggie. *Intimate Partners: Patterns in Love and Marriage.* New York: Random House, 1987.

Schaef, Anne Wilson. *Co-dependence: Misunderstood—Mistreated.* Minneapolis: Winston Press, 1986.

Scheingold, L.D., and N. Wagner. *Sound Sex and the Aging Heart.* New York: Human Sciences Press, 1974.

Schover, Leslie. *Prime Time: Sexual Health for Men Over Fifty.* New York: Holt, Rinehart & Winston, 1984.

Scott-Maxwell, Florida. *The Measure of My Days.* New York: Penguin Books, 1979.

Selye, Hans, M.D. The *Stress of Life.* New York: McGraw-Hill Book Co., 1956.

Shbayama, Abbot Zenkei. *A Flower Does Not Talk.* Rutland, Vt., and Tokyo, Japan: Charles E. Tuttle Co., 1970.

Sheehy, Gail. *Passages.* New York: E.P. Dutton & Co., 1976.

Shneidman, Edwin S. *Deaths of Man.* Baltimore: Penguin Books, 1973.

Simonton, O.C., S. Simonton, and J. Creighton. *Getting Well Again.* Los Angeles: J.P. Tarcher, 1978.

Smedes, Lewis B. *Forgive and Forget: Healing the Hurts We Don't Deserve.* San Francisco: Harper & Row, 1984.

Sotile, Wayne M., Ph.D. *Heart Illness and Intimacy, How Caring Relationships Aid Recovery.* Baltimore: The Johns Hopkins University Press, 1992.

Speedling, Edward J. *Heart Attack: The Family Response at Home and in the Hospital.* New York: Tavistock Publications, 1982.

Stauffer, Edith R., Ph.D. *Unconditional Love and Forgiveness.* Burbank, Calif.: Triangle Publishers, 1987.

Stern, Ellen Sue. *Expecting Change.* New York: Poseidon Press, 1986.

Strong, Maggie. *Mainstay: For the Well Spouse of the Chronically Ill.* Boston: Little, Brown & Co., 1988.

Tatelbaum, Judy. *The Courage to Grieve.* New York: Perennial Library, Harper & Row, 1980.

Veninga, Robert. *A Gift of Hope: How We Survive Our Tragedies.* Boston: Little, Brown & Co., 1985.

Viorst, Judith. *Necessary Losses.* New York: Fawcett Gold Medal, 1986.

Viscott, David, M.D. *How To Live With Another Person.* New York: Pocket Books, 1974.

———. *The Language of Feelings.* New York: Pocket Books, 1976.

Waxberg, Joseph D., M.D. *Bypass: A Doctor's Recovery from Open Heart Surgery.* New York: Appleton-Century-Crofts, 1981.

Wilber, Ken. *Eye to Eye.* New York: Anchor Books, 1983.

INDEX

241

Heartmates® is an ongoing therapeutic program designed to serve the cardiac spouse and family during and after a cardiac crisis. To be included on our mailing list, please print your name and address below and mail to:

Heartmates, Inc.
P.O. Box 16202
Minneapolis, MN 55416
USA

Or share your questions and concerns with us via e-mail:

heartmates@aol.com

Your age now: ——————— Your spouse's age: ———————
Date of onset of heart disease: ————————————————
What has changed most in *your* life since the onset of your mate's heart disease? ————————————————————————

————————————————————————————————————

What concerns you most right now? ————————————————

————————————————————————————————————

TO ORDER PERSONAL HEARTMATES® RESOURCES...

A Videoseries, *Portrait of a Heartmate*; each of five-20 minute programs focuses on a different topic. Titles are: *"After A Heart Attack," "Understanding Cardiac Care," "The Road To Recovery," "Family Concerns,"* and *"Renewing The Relationship."* This series is available for personal use and costs US $59.95, including shipping and handling.

A new interactive and user-friendly resource; *The Heartmates® Meditation Journal: A Daily Companion for Partners of Heart Patients.* This yearlong aid focuses on the changes in the heartmate's life when a partner has heart disease. A beautiful edition, *The Heartmates Meditation Journal* makes a wonderful gift and will fit in purse or briefcase...a support companion you will want to use daily. US $15.00, including shipping and handling.

Heartmates® Inc. will accept personal checks in US funds, or will charge your order to your...
❏ VISA – or – ❏ MASTERCARD
Your card number: ————————————————
Expiration date: ————————————————
❏ Portrait of a Heartmate Videoseries
❏ The Heartmates® Meditation Journal: A Daily Companion

NAME ——————————————————————————————

ADDRESS ————————————————————————————

CITY———————————————— PROV. ———————————

POSTAL ZONE———————————— PHONE (———) ——————

Heartmates® is an ongoing therapeutic program designed to serve the cardiac spouse and family during and after a cardiac crisis. To be included on our mailing list, please print your name and address below and mail to:

Heartmates, Inc.
P.O. Box 16202
Minneapolis, MN 55416
USA

Or share your questions and concerns with us via e-mail:

heartmates@aol.com

Your age now: _____ Your spouse's age: _____
Date of onset of heart disease: _____
What has changed most in *your* life since the onset of your mate's heart disease? _____

_____

What concerns you most right now? _____

_____

TO ORDER PERSONAL HEARTMATES® RESOURCES...

A Videoseries, *Portrait of a Heartmate*; each of five-20 minute programs focuses on a different topic. Titles are: *"After A Heart Attack," "Understanding Cardiac Care," "The Road To Recovery," "Family Concerns," and "Renewing The Relationship."* This series is available for personal use and costs US $59.95, including shipping and handling.

A new interactive and user-friendly resource; *The Heartmates® Meditation Journal: A Daily Companion for Partners of Heart Patients.* This yearlong aid focuses on the changes in the heartmate's life when a partner has heart disease. A beautiful edition, *The Heartmates Meditation Journal* makes a wonderful gift and will fit in purse or briefcase...a support companion you will want to use daily. US $15.00, including shipping and handling.

Heartmates® Inc. will accept personal checks in US funds, or will charge your order to your...
        ❏ VISA – or – ❏ MASTERCARD
    Your card number: _____
    Expiration date: _____
❏ Portrait of a Heartmate Videoseries
❏ The Heartmates® Meditation Journal: A Daily Companion

NAME _____

ADDRESS _____

CITY_____ PROV. _____

POSTAL ZONE_____ PHONE (____) _____